Brain Attack

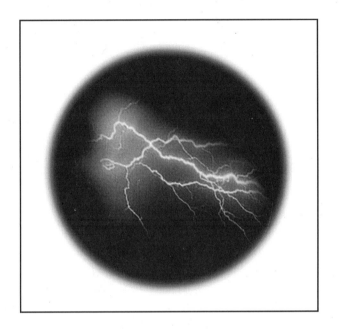

Danger

Chaos

Opportunity

Empowerment

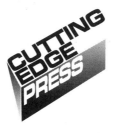

A division of Perez Enterprises, Inc.
287 Whiteface Mountain Dr.
Johnson, Vermont 05656

▾

Printed in the United States

Book and Cover Design by Jim Fitzgerald
Edited by Marsha Rehns

II

The author acknowledges permission to reprint the following:

The Stroke Survivor Bill of Rights, Excerpted from *Out of the Blue: One Woman's Story of Stroke, Love and Survival* by Bonnie Sherr Klein, copyright 1999, Wildcat Canyon Press.

Library of Congress Cataloging in Publication Data

Paulina G. Perez

Brain Attack: Danger, Chaos, Opportunity, and Empowerment

by Paulina Perez,

foreword by Robert Scaer M.D.

Library of Congress Catalogue Number 2001 126348

ISBN 0-9641159-5-6

1. Stroke–popular work

2. Brain Attack– Psychology

3. Aphasia–rehabilitation

4. Title

The quotations that precede each entry in this book empowered me while I recovered from the brain attack and learned to speak again. The words of others inspired me throughout the year after the stroke and helped me tap into the determination, pluck, and courage that I didn't know I had deep inside of me.

Brain Attack

Table of Contents

Foreword V
Acknowledgments IX
Introduction XII

Part One

Chapter One: The First Day 1
Chapter Two: I Can Spot Excellence Quickly 27
Chapter Three: On with My Life 47
Chapter Four: The Start of the Last Year of the Century 53
Chapter Five: Sink or Swim 61
Chapter Six: My War with Words 73
Chapter Seven: Soul Searching 89
Chapter Eight: Ambitious Goals 103
Chapter Nine: Spring Brings New Life 121
Chapter Ten: First Professional Speech 135
Chapter Eleven: Facing Adversity 151
Chapter Twelve: I Need a Break 159
Chapter Thirteen: Cutting the Cord 169
Chapter Fourteen: Trying to Be a Nurse Again 181
Chapter Fifteen: Pure Fear 195
Chapter Sixteen: Better than Last Year 209
Chapter Seventeen: My Saints 220
Chapter Eighteen: When we're ready to learn the lesson,
                      the teacher will appear. 221

Part Two

Revamping Attitudes Toward Health Care: From a Nurse's Perspective 225
Revamping Attitudes Toward Health Care: From a Patient's Perspective 228
Don't Step on My Courage 228
A Word to My Fellow Survivors 229
Family-Centered Stroke Care 230
Principles of Family-Centered Care 231
Stroke Survivor/ Family/ Professional Collaboration 231
Tips about Aphasia for Family and Friends 232

Appendix

The Effects of a Stroke 233
Stroke Survivors 234
Types of Brain Attack 235
Aphasia: Where Have My Words Gone? 236
Resources 238
Internet Resources 241
Stroke Survivor's Bill of Rights 242
Glossary 243
Bibliography 247

Foreword

Stroke—the familiar term for what physicians call a cerebral infarct— conveys the shock, terror, helplessness, and irrevocable life change that characterize this common clinical event. In contrast to the course of most human illnesses, the full expression of a stroke occurs within seconds or minutes, suddenly depriving victims of the most basic functions of daily life. Swallowing, smiling, sight, speech, comprehension, thinking, feeling, moving become by virtue of their loss the stroke victim's most precious possessions. Stroke survivors would give away any portion of their worldly possessions to restore at least part of these "simple" functions that healthy people take for granted. A stroke typically steals a piece of what can be described only as the self—the perception of one's own intrinsic meaning and worth.

As a practicing neurologist who has treated and helped rehabilitated thousands of stroke patients, I feel that I have seen virtually every possible combination of neurologic deficits attributable to a cerebral infarct. I have a keen sense of the suffering many stroke victims face on the road back to functioning. Yet I would not presume to understand the pain, frustration, and despair that this long and arduous process can provoke. Strokes often seem to have a way of interrupting those functions most precious to the victim: aphasia in an author and public speaker like Polly Perez, for example. Physical disabilities apparent to others are not necessarily the most frustrating disabilities stroke victims face. More frightening are subtle or not-so-subtle changes in perception, thinking, and regulation of emotions. In many cases these strange and startling cognitive changes challenge victims' sense of wholeness, their sense of survival of the self.

In her book, Polly Perez vividly describes her feeling of being trapped in her own body, a body that no longer responded to the most basic command and a mind that failed to formulate the most simple thought in words. Her vivid description of riding a terrifying emotional roller coaster during her stroke is also a seldom-described but common accompaniment to a cerebral infarct. One function of the cerebral cortex is to regulate and modify the more primitive emotional functions of the brain. Loss of even a portion of cortical function in a stroke often leads to distressing and uncontrollable emotional lability, which may be perplexing and at times embarrassing. Tears may flow at the slightest sentimental thought or image. Helpless rage may erupt over trivial frustrations. Fortunately, this emotional deficit often is one of the earliest to improve.

The quality of recovery from a stroke depends on many factors. The early use of blood-clot inhibitors such as tPA represents a new, aggressive, and exciting development. Despite their risks, these inhibitors appear to offer our first real chance of altering and at times reversing the progression of brain damage in a stroke. Safer variations of tPA can be expected. In the long run, however, I have found that stroke victims' strength of character may be the secret element in their recovery.

We used to believe that we are endowed with a fixed brain structure and number of brain cells. Recent neurologic research has demonstrated, however, that experience alters our brains chemically and even structurally. The current concept that rehabilitation, such as the speech therapy that Polly Perez received, serves only to maximize what brain function is left, may be replaced by concepts of training-induced formation of new brain cells and pathways. If so, then determination, fortitude, and endless repetition may be the key to optimal stroke recovery. There may be no fixed timeline when therapeutic retraining of the stroke victim is no longer of use. The progress of brain alteration and restructuring through training may lead to new behavioral techniques in stroke rehabilitation.

This book is about more than the intimate and personal journey of a stroke victim to recovery and perhaps redemption. Also in the text are recurrent and disturbing references to a flawed system of delivery of medical care. The comments are similar to those I have heard from dozens of patients about their experience in our hospital system. But the observations in this book were made by a nurse, which lends them objectivity and accuracy. Any life-threatening experience such as a stroke or major surgery is traumatizing and life-changing. Patients are helpless and vulnerable, totally dependent on their caregivers. Patients' families face a similar potential for traumatic loss. Under such conditions, anger toward patients or rejection of their needs by caregivers is virtually certain to be perceived far more intensely by the patient and their families than in less-stressful situations.

Most doctors and psychiatrists have ignored the emotional trauma associated with a life-threatening illness, the machines used in diagnosis, and the often painful and terrifying treatment. Studies of the incidence of posttraumatic stress disorder in cancer and heart surgery survivors have only recently been published. Even studies investigating the psychological effects of awakening under anesthesia, an event that occurs more than 30,000 times each year, have been limited to a handful. The results of these studies suggest a shocking incidence of long-term emotional disturbance in patients with critical illness, related in many instances not only to the disease, but also to the attitude and demeanor of caregivers. In the stroke patient, whose perception and communication may be distorted or impaired, the perception and communication that remain are often sensitized and acute. In such instances, shaking of the head, grimacing, or frowning by a nurse at an aphasic patient's attempts at speech can be devastating. Somehow we in the healing professions must rediscover the principles of empathic caring within the whirlwind of lifesaving technology.

Few stroke survivors have the strength or facility to look within themselves for insights they might gain from their loss. This book represents a unique effort by a writer and also a unique opportunity for readers to understand the deepest thoughts and feelings of a stroke survivor. In my practice I've seen that even family members have great difficulty understanding the stroke patient's behavior. They often feel that the person they love is no longer there. Stroke victims' inability to express their thoughts accurately places a seemingly impenetrable barrier between them and those around them. The obvious distress of family members adds to the patient's despair and frustration. The insights that Polly Perez reached during her long recovery offer a ray of light and understanding to the families of stroke survivors, allowing them to empathize with their loved one's trials and to realize that the cherished person is still there. Stroke survivors who read this book will be fortified by the realization that others have faced the same sense of irreparable loss and not only survived, but thrived.

Members of the healing professions would also be well served by studying Polly Perez's odyssey. I wish every physician would read this book and assimilate the sense of loss that can arise in patients who perceive dismissal and rejection from their caregivers. I wish every nurse would realize the profound effect that a negative expression or critical word has on their vulnerable and helpless patients. But even those caregivers with the most noble and caring intentions would benefit from the insights derived in Polly Perez's amazing journal. This is an essential book for rehabilitation therapists, nurses, counselors, and physicians at all levels of training.

Occasionally, fortuitously, adversity gives rise to deliverance and transformation. It may be that we can understand the value of our existence only through loss or threatened loss. Severe disability may bring life into much clearer focus, as many cancer survivors know. In stroke patients, however, a dauntless force of will often seems necessary to achieve this deeper understanding along with an acceptance that recovery requires a lifelong commitment. A stroke survivor who views her brain attack as an opportunity and potential source of empowerment has already traveled half the journey.

Robert Scaer, M.D.
Neurologist
Medical Director, Retired
Mapleton Rehabilitation Center

Brain Attack

For Jane and Donna, my lifelines

<u>To Jane</u>

*After the verb 'to Love,' 'to Help' is the most
beautiful verb in the world.*

Bertha von Suttner

You are my unrecognized hero and are family and friend rolled into one. By your advocacy efforts, you led me out of the wilderness and shadows and back into the light and speaking world once again. Without you, I would have been lost in a wordless world.

<u>To Donna</u>

*In a garden, we do not 'grow' flowers,
we create the conditions in which flowers can grow.*

Ram Dass

I'm thankful that life let me stumble onto you. I love how big your heart is. After the stroke, your trust in me spoke volumes when I couldn't speak. My speaking life was in your hands, and you kept it safe until I learned to speak again.

Acknowledgments

A sound ship needs a course to follow,
no matter what the condition is on the sea.

To Eric

A life without love is like a sunless garden
when the flowers are dead.
The consciousness of loving and being loved brings a warmth
and richness to life that nothing else can bring.

Oscar Wilde

You are the person who kept me going with your unconditional support. Every time I asked you, "Do you think that I will be able to be a public speaker again?" you said, "Sure," and meant it. I drew on your strength and belief that I would do professional public speaking again. Thank you for being there through thick and thin for the last 35 years.

To Marsha

Writing is an adventure.
To begin with, it is a toy and an amusement.
Then it becomes a mistress,
then it becomes a master,
then it becomes a tyrant.
The last phase is that just as you are to be reconciled
to your servitude,
you kill the monster and fling him to the public.

Winston Churchill

You were pivotal in the publication of this book. The fact that you believed in it and in my ability to write it gave me hope as I put my fractured words on paper. Your patience in making sense of my grammar as I relearned to spell and write was critical and your amazing talents as an editor gave this book life.

To Jean

Do the right thing.

It will gratify some people and astonish the rest.

Mark Twain

We are a good match as we both have feisty spirits. I was lucky to find a doctor like you that followed her instincts and her heart. You took a risk when you gave me tPA but by doing that you gave me a fighting chance to recover my life.

To Marje

How beautiful a day can be when kindness touches it.

George Elliston

Seeing your shining face in the ER while confusion reigned around me gave me hope. Your calm strength helped me more than you will ever know. Thanks for advocating for me and taking a risk when I needed to change hospitals. You have a heart of gold.

To Debbie

And we find at the end of the perfect day,
the soul of a friend we've made.

Carrie Jacobs Bond

We locked spirits immediately, and I gravitated instantly to your great natural warmth. I was right in fighting to work with you, as you had faith in me when I had none.

To Steve

He deserves paradise who makes his companions laugh.

The Koran

You did an amazing job of balancing your time in teaching, encouraging, and supporting me. Your sense of humor made some of my darkest days bearable.

To my family, friends, and colleagues

The love we give away is the only love we keep.

Elbert Hubbard

All of you have been an important part of a nourishing partnership that I needed in order to recover my life.

Introduction

When nothing is sure, everything is possible.
Margaret Drabble

Life can have a way of sneaking up on you and knocking you off balance. A stroke does just that. It is the number one cause of adult disability in the United States, killing 150,000 Americans every year and throwing the lives of another 350,000 into chaos. Someone in this country suffers a brain attack every 53 seconds, and four out of five American families will be affected by this tumultuous event.

Men have strokes more often than women do, but more women die from strokes, possibly because they are more likely to be older and to live alone at the time of the brain attack than men are. Strokes kill about 90,000 women every year–more than twice as many women as die from breast cancer.

I am a 54-year-old nurse and lecturer, and I am a survivor of a brain attack. I don't know what caused my stroke, which is not unusual–40 percent of strokes are unexplained. The most common risk factors for stroke are hypertension (high blood pressure), heart disease, atrial fibrillation (irregular heartbeat), a previous stroke, a previous ministroke called a transient ischemic attack (TIA), and cigarette smoking. I had none of those risk factors, although ten years ago I had an episode of dizziness and double vision that was never diagnosed as a stroke or TIA. In retrospect, it may have been a minor stroke.

The stroke I had on an ordinary December morning was sudden and unexpected, and the blood clots in my brain jumbled not only my thoughts but also my life. The damage to the neurological connections in my brain presented me with unique challenges and dilemmas as well as with unique opportunities.

The language center of my brain suffered the greatest damage. I am now one of the one million people in the United States who have aphasia (uh-fay'-zhuh) and apraxia (uh-prax'-ee-a) as the result of surviving a stroke. Aphasia is an inability to articulate words. Apraxia is an inability to perform a well-known purposeful action in spite of having normal mobility, attention, and comprehension. I know the word I want to say, but by the time the word reaches my lips, it has changed in whole or in part to something else.

The severity of aphasia and apraxia can range from mild to severe. My apraxia and aphasia were severe, and they forced me to change the way that I communicated. Before the stroke I was a public speaker, so spoken language was my life. Not being able to speak was sheer terror. There is no cure for aphasia, but it can be treated and ameliorated with speech therapy. Wresting my speech back was the hardest thing I have ever done.

Like many people who have aphasia, I also had weakness on my right side. The two deficits went together because the stroke damaged the left side of my brain, which directs the right side of the body and also many aspects of speech.

I want you to read how it feels when your world changes, and the things that were on the bottom are on top. My words were abducted, and a life without words altered my perception of reality. Think of what it would be like to have stripped away from you the simplest capabilities that you take for granted, like writing, talking, or even adding up a check at a restaurant. I wasn't stupid; I just had difficulty saying words. I could read, but I couldn't write. I wasn't mindless, just wordless. I wasn't uneducated, but I couldn't talk right. My identity was more than what I could say; inside I was the same person that I was before the stroke.

The stroke was a cruel, random attack from which I emerged sorely damaged. A shock surrounded me, and I felt separate from others. Words were in my head, but I couldn't get them out. People spoke at me, not with me.

I must say, though, that as I recovered from the brain attack, I was never bored. Each day I unearthed things that I had to learn again. I often wept out of frustration, but I kept going anyway. I accepted the challenge of speaking again. I discovered a capacity for courage and endurance that I hadn't known. My self-esteem and my determination survived.

This tale of loss, determination, and discovery describes my feelings, my fears, my emotional pain, and my hopes as I traveled the rough road away from my brain attack. I want people to realize that the stroke didn't change my soul.

Writing about feelings is intensely personal. The feelings that we stroke survivors have deep inside of us are meaningful, and our friends and families need to understand them. The understanding of health-care providers is especially important. If they are willing to make the effort, health-care workers can give a voice to those of us who have lost ours. I want to know who in the health-care system is listening to the messages in the hearts of stroke victims. Nurses? I want to know who is listening to our hopes. Doctors? I want to know who is listening to our fears. Physical therapists and occupational therapists? I want to know who is listening to our dreams. Speech therapists? All these professionals were involved in my search for wellness and fluent speech.

Stroke survivors and health-care worker alike can feel helpless and hopeless when faced with the ravages of brain attacks, and it's easy for health-care professionals to think of people who have had a brain attack as a collection of symptoms instead of as feeling, thinking human beings. But if nurses, doctors. occupational therapists, physical therapists, speech therapists, and speech pathologists are to help stroke victims, they need to recognize how drastically the life of the stroke victim changes. In health care, some decisions are made in the head, but they should be made in the heart too.

I invite readers to experience through this book how it feels to have a brain attack, aphasia, and apraxia. If you face a difficult passage in this book, please stay with it; it will help you appreciate what stroke survivors endure. If you feel emotional, savor the feeling; it will help you know how to help us.

I labored a long time to write this book. What you read came from my heart and soul. I needed to put my feelings onto the page so they didn't overwhelm me. At first, it was hard to call up the words that I wanted to write, and I kept note cards around my house so that whenever the right phrase or words came into my mind I could write them down. I have written four books before, but writing this one was much harder. I tried to write honestly, insightfully, and truthfully about the agony of strokes, apraxia, and aphasia. I recorded the meaningful things that happened to me for the first year after the brain attack as I went through physical, occupational, and speech therapy. This book reveals the deepest texture of my soul. It is about strokes and the health-care system but also about issues of the heart.

Read my story, and step through the doorway of a stroke victim's life. Journey with me through the changes a brain attack victim faces. You will find, as I did, that there are many intense physical and emotional feelings ahead. Experience the feelings and honor them. Those of us who were damaged by a brain malady have had to do just that.

Chapter One
The First Day

It is a relief when things get to their worst.
You know what the worst is and can begin to plan better.
Elinore Pruitt Stewart

I never envisioned anything like a brain attack when December 1998 started. My life had already changed enough. I had recently left Houston, the city I had called home for 35 years, and settled down to a quieter life in rural Vermont. I had been home for three days from a speaking engagement in Florida, and I was looking forward to the end of the year. Instead, a thunderbolt to my brain stole my life from me. The brain attack was like a sudden dive into a vast, dark sea.

December 9, 1998

In choosing the beginning of a road,
we also choose its destination.
A folk saying

The day was normal in most respects when I got on my treadmill, as I did most mornings, to take a five-mile walk. I watched television for distraction. When I was almost finished walking, I noticed I could barely hear the television. My first reaction was that I needed to turn up the sound. That moment marked the end of the life I had known and the start of my journey through the kingdom of the unwell. I knew that I was on my treadmill in my house, I was aware of the treadmill moving under my feet, but nothing else seemed right. Something was drastically wrong.

Coherent thoughts refused to form in my mind. I am usually good about listening to my body, but it wasn't telling me anything. I felt as if I was staring at a blank page. One question kept forming in my mind: "What went wrong?" I tried to understand what was happening. Everything inside me felt like it was being pulled down. I maneuvered my legs to the sides of the treadmill frame, off the moving belt. I tried to pull the key out, but I couldn't. I felt an other-worldliness, and I realized that I wasn't thinking clearly. I seemed to be caught by an all-encompassing force that was more powerful than my thoughts. I sensed an extraordinary upheaval in my brain, but I couldn't explain it to myself. I was different and I knew it, yet I couldn't understand what was going on.

My thoughts seemed to be slipping away, and I tried to hold on to them. I tried to grasp any idea at all but to no avail. I clawed at my thoughts as a cat does with a piece of wood. I thumbed through my brain as you would do with a Rolodex file, but I was bewildered by possibilities. It was odd, but I never felt helpless, even though I knew that a storm had invaded my brain and my being. I didn't have time to be apprehensive or afraid. It seemed that someone was looking for me. I ignored the call until I couldn't ignore it any longer. Who was calling? My brain seemed muddled, and I had trouble understanding what to do. I felt like I was fading away, but I had a problem to solve before I left. How could I get someone to help me?

I yelled for my husband, Eric, but he seemed not to hear me. "I'm in plain trouble here," I thought to myself. I was afraid to let go of the bar of the treadmill, but I knew I needed to do that in order to get the key out of the machine and turn it off. I tried to devise a plan to escape from the exercise machine, even though I was still having trouble thinking. It took three tries to get enough confidence to pull the key out. When I finally got it out, I felt like saying "Yes!" with my arms raised in celebration.

MEDICAL FACTS

The warning signs of a stroke include the following:

- Numbness or weakness in the face, an arm, or a leg
- Difficulty speaking or understanding
- Difficulty swallowing
- Severe headache
- Sudden confusion
- Dizziness or loss of balance
- Sudden blurred or decreased vision
- Sudden change in mental ability

National Stroke Association

Fear knocked at the door. Faith answered, and no one was there.

My life was unraveling thread by thread like a piece of cloth. I yelled again for Eric, but he still didn't seem to hear me. I tried to signal him that I was in distress. I banged on the treadmill with my left hand and told myself that I must not panic. I tried to think of what else I could do. I was still holding on to the treadmill and yelling, "Help!" At least I thought I was yelling, "Help!" Nothing worked. As I knew I had to save myself, I didn't have time to be anxious. I have always believed in my ability to meet the challenges in my life. I thought to myself, "I'm really in a pickle now, but I'll do my best with this situation." I kept trying to think how I could get someone to answer me or help me. Then I began to be aware that something was wrong with my right side. I knew that I needed to get off the treadmill. I tried to walk, but my right leg abandoned me. I couldn't move it as I used to, so I finally decided that the best thing to do was to fall down. I landed on the floor by the treadmill, and I focused my energy on crawling inch by inch to the hallway. That's where Eric found me.

He kept asking me what I wanted to do. I kept answering him, but he didn't seem to understand what I was saying. He finally asked me if I was saying to call an ambulance, and I nodded, "Yes." It seemed to me that I was a free-floating presence–neither here nor there. I had no idea what lay ahead of me. Eric called an ambulance and my sister-in-law, Jane, who is a nurse. She and my brother, Michael, would meet us at the local hospital.

As Eric was talking to 911, the nurse in me took over. I knew that the paramedics would never get up our narrow stairs with a stretcher, so I bumped down the stairs step by step on my backside even though part of my right side was not working well. I was always aware of what was happening around me. I knew that I needed to have my insurance card to get into the hospital, so I crawled on my hands and knees into my living room to get my purse. I couldn't figure out which card was the insurance one because the letters on the cards held no meaning for me, as if they were in a foreign language. I found the insurance card by remembering what color it was. When Eric found me, I was clutching the card in my hand.

In the ambulance, the emergency medical technician speculated that I was sick because I had been exercising and my blood sugar was low. I thought to myself, "This is worse than low blood sugar." I felt numb inside, but I also had an amazing sense of calm. In the recesses of my nurse-trained mind,

Brain Attack

I knew that in the emergency room (ER) they would tell me I had had a stroke. I felt that I had been left on the shore of an ocean. As waves lapped around me, I worried that the tide would carry me under.

Jane was waiting for me when I arrived at the ER in Copley Hospital. Copley is a small, old, two-story hospital in another town about nine miles away. Jane held my hand. This smallest of gestures was a pure expression of love and one I needed mightily. I am tough on the outside but sometimes quite vulnerable inside. This was one of the vulnerable times. I felt as if I was floating even though I knew I was on a bed. Jane's gentle hand seemed to anchor me so I wouldn't float away.

The word "surrender" evokes giving up and giving in, and this was not what I wanted to do. But I had been dumped into the middle of a maelstrom, and confusion reigned around me. I surrendered to the sensations going on in my brain.

MEDICAL FACTS

In the emergency room (ER), an evaluation is done to confirm that the source of the patient's problem is a stroke. One aim of emergency care is to determine the most likely causes of the stroke. Another aim is to predict the likelihood of immediate complications. A third goal is to begin appropriate treatment.

The following happens when a person enters the ER with a suspected stroke:

- Staff members immediately connect the patient to equipment to monitor heart rate, blood pressure, and level of oxygen in the blood.
- Oxygen is given through the nose.
- A quick history and physical are completed, and the time the stroke occurred is determined
- A neurological exam is performed.
- Blood is drawn.
- An electrocardiogram (EKG) is performed.
- Intravenous lines are started to deliver fluids and medications.
- A computerized axial tomography (CAT) scan of the brain is completed.

A brain attack occurs when blood circulation to the brain fails, and brain cells die from the resulting lack of oxygen. Strokes are classified into two categories: those that are caused by a blockage of a blood vessel, which is called ischemia, and those caused by bleeding inside the brain, called a hemorrhagic stroke.

Four-fifths of strokes are the result of ischemia. Blockage of a blood vessel has three major causes: the formation of a blood clot within a blood vessel of the brain or neck (thrombosis), the movement to the brain of a clot formed in another part of the body (embolism); or a severe narrowing of an artery in or leading to the brain (stenosis).

Clinical studies suggest that thrombolytic (anti-clotting) drugs given within a few hours after the start of an ischemic stroke may significantly limit the extent of brain injury and may not be complicated by the high rates of hemorrhage that physicians originally feared.

Stroke Council--American Heart Association

I was puzzled as to why the doctor in the ER didn't tell me anything about my condition. I found out later that he was telling my family that I had suffered a stroke. I wish he had told me first. Even if he thought I couldn't understand or hear clearly, he should have paid me the respect of communicating to me that I had had a brain attack. After all, it was my life that had abruptly changed.

The ER doctor told us nothing about treating strokes with tissue plasminogen activator (tPA). I had known about tPA, a drug that can break up the clots that block the flow of blood to the brain and cause a stroke, and I couldn't understand why I wasn't getting it. To be effective, tPA must be given within three hours of the brain attack. In my mind, I was asking questions: Why weren't they talking to me? Didn't they understand me? Were they ignoring me on purpose? Why weren't they listening to me?

I was fortunate that more than once my sister-in-law asked the right questions. The ER doctor told her that tPA was an experimental drug (which is not true), but she kept asking about my getting it. She kept after the doctor until he called a neurologist at a regional medical center in Burlington and another on the Copley staff. The local neurologist ordered a CAT scan of my brain, determined that I wasn't bleeding there (tPA can make a hemorrhagic stroke worse), and concluded that I was, in medical jargon, a good candidate for tPA.

The neurologist in that small hospital understood what I needed. The tPA would prevent further damage to the area of my brain that controls speech, but it had to be given within three hours after I had the stroke, and time was running out.

Jane told the doctors that they had to talk to me about the drug's risks and benefits. When the doctors, Jane, and Eric entered the ER from the waiting room, Eric looked sad and confused. The neurologist told me about the risks, and Jane asked me if I understood. I did understand what they were saying, and I told them "yes" and "no" by moving my head. I was the one that would remain the same, get better, or die, and I wanted to be the one to make the decision. I have more than a touch of fighter and risk-taker in me, and I decided that I wanted to risk taking the drug. I was so glad that Jane was there and

5

argued on my behalf. The tPA was given to me intravenously, but because of the possibility that the drug could cause bleeding in my brain, I had to be transferred to the medical center hospital in case I needed to be treated for hemorrhaging.

MEDICAL FACTS

Since 1996, when the Food and Drug Administration approved tissue plasminogen activator (tPA) to treat stroke, thousands of people have received the drug. The potentially lifesaving medication can be given safely to stroke patients at small hospitals in rural areas and small towns, not just at major medical centers with stroke specialists on staff.

Stroke 2000, 31.

In the ER, I thought that I was speaking normally. I didn't realize that I was saying the same word over and over, and I couldn't understand why people weren't communicating with me. They talked to everyone except me. No one told me that although I was talking a lot, the words I thought I was saying weren't words at all–just sounds that didn't even resemble words. It seemed that my speech had exploded; words were scattered everywhere, and I couldn't find them.

The day had its own momentum. I couldn't trust my senses or myself.

I had been in the ER a little more than two hours when my friend Marje, who is also a nurse, came in. I didn't know how she knew that I was there, but she was a balm for my soul. Her smile gave me hope, as I felt her protective hand on my left arm. I was glad to have two good advocates who cared about me.

The tone in the ER was serious, and I could see it reflected on Eric's, Jane's, and Michael's faces. Eric looked lost, and I was glad that Jane was there to support him as well as me. As the emergency medical technicians (EMTs) were putting me into the ambulance for the transfer to the medical center, they asked me whom I wanted to ride with me in the ambulance. The answer was easy. Jane was my lifeline. I knew that she would protect my interests. I nodded my head and pointed to her. Jane rode in the back of the ambulance with me, but I couldn't see her, so I thought she was up front. I felt utterly alone, even though the EMTs were monitoring my vital signs. I was too sick to be the warrior I usually am, so this job was relegated to Jane. I needed her with me. I knew that she would love me, nurture me, and shield me from harm.

Just before I left the ER, the neurologist gave Eric her office and home telephone numbers and told him that he could call her. We couldn't know then how grateful we would be for that courtesy.

I arrived at the medical center at about 11 am. I was taken to the intensive care unit (ICU), where I was hooked up to what seemed to be every conceivable wire and tube. The heart monitor over my head beeped incessantly. The beeping pecked away at my brain, and I tried to shut it out by slipping into slumber.

I found that many times I was treated as if I wasn't there. Already I didn't like it when people ignored me and talked around me as if I couldn't understand. I knew what was happening; I just couldn't say anything. Jane was the only person who understood that I had to be consulted about everything.

Jane stayed with me all that day and all night. I knew that the nurses in the ICU were good because they understood that I needed to have Jane with me. They never treated her like an intruder but like an important member of my health-care team. Jane was the first person who talked slowly enough for me to understand what was being said.

The truth began to dawn on me that what I was saying was gibberish. The words that I wanted to say had disappeared. What I was trying to say sounded to others like nonsense. Conversations were one-sided. My desire to say a word was overwhelming, but most of the time nothing came out. Words seemed to have gotten misplaced in my head, skittering behind closed doors in my mind. Surprisingly, Jane and I giggled, laughed, and guffawed about my attempts to say words. We laughed so much that we worried that the nurses might come in and tell us to stop making a ruckus. There in the middle of ICU, with my brain scrambled, I found levity in a bleak scene. Together, Jane and I used the learn-as-you-go method to communicate. We used pantomime, questions from her, and nods and gestures from me–anything that got the idea across.

The day was endless. My existence seemed to be stretched over time like plastic wrap. I could see what was in my life, but I couldn't feel it. I still couldn't hear very well. My hearing kept diminishing as if someone had turned down a rheostat, but looking at the person talking to me helped my comprehension.

The realization that Jane and the drug tPA had stopped my free fall into a world without words overcame me. I knew that I had scores of challenges ahead. This feisty, plain-spoken woman was ready for a fight.

MEDICAL FACTS

A brain attack is a sudden loss of movement, sensation, vision, speech and/or thinking ability due to the death or injury of nerve cells in the brain.

The left hemisphere of the brain controls the movement of the right side of the body. It also controls speech and language abilities. Someone who has a left-hemisphere brain attack may develop aphasia.

Stroke Council--American Heart Association

FROM THE NEUROLOGIST

I was called from my office to see a new patient in the ER whose family had asked for a neurology consult. My first impression was of a woman with panic in her eyes. I immediately felt a sense of connection to her. Here was another health-care professional who knew about doctors and hospitals but couldn't speak. She was someone from "my" world who was on the other side of health care.

After my initial evaluation, I knew that Polly was a good candidate for tPA. I practice in a 50-bed hospital in a rural community, and I don't have other neurology colleagues to bounce ideas off of. I was told by those in a tertiary-care [more sophisticated] hospital to send her to them in an ambulance. They told me not to use tPA in our hospital, but I felt the drug was Polly's best option. I thought that she would want to take it and accept the accompanying risks. I sensed Polly's frantic response to the stroke and aphasia, and I was determined that she would get the tPA.

This was only my second experience with tPA, and I was feeling a sense of inadequacy. We were nearing the three-hour limit for giving the drug, and I was pressured and nervous. I was unhappy about sending Polly to another hospital after making the initial evaluation and treatment choices, but because of the potential side effects of tPA, I was forced to transfer Polly to the medical center. Not wanting her to get lost in the large, impersonal institution, I gave my home phone number to her husband and sister-in-law so I could maintain contact with them. My calls to the neurology service at the medical center hospital were not returned, so I kept tabs on Polly through her sister-in-law, Jane.

Eric

I knew something was wrong when I found Polly in the hall on her hands and knees, making no sense when she spoke. When I asked her if I should call an ambulance and she nodded, "Yes" I knew that she was in bad shape, as Polly rarely concedes that she needs medical attention for anything.

While I was calling the ambulance and then her brother and sister-in-law, Mike and Jane, Polly had gotten herself down the stairs and was going through her purse. I asked her what she was doing, and she answered, "Brank." I figured out that she was looking for her insurance card, since she knew that she would need it to get into the hospital. I felt less scared because I knew that she understood what was going on around her. She just couldn't talk.

Jane and Mike were at the hospital when we arrived, and I knew that since Jane was a nurse, she could tell me what was going on. I could tell from Polly's eyes that she knew what was happening too, and I felt better knowing that Polly could make a decision about whatever the doctor in the ER wanted to do. I remembered seeing something on television in Houston about a drug that should be given within the first few hours after a stroke. I didn't know what the drug was called, but Jane knew it was tPA. She kept questioning the emergency room doctor about administering it. We asked Polly about giving her tPA, and she nodded her head. The ER doctor got the drug after the neurologist at the hospital said that Polly would be a perfect candidate for it.

I felt relieved. I was glad that Jane was going with Polly in the ambulance to the medical center. I knew that if anything happened on the way Polly would have with her someone who would do anything to save her.

I knew that Polly was going to be all right because she understood everything I was telling her and she hadn't lost her ability to think. Knowing Polly as I do, I knew that she would dedicate all her energy to getting better. If anyone could do it, she would.

Jane

Polly and I had been professional colleagues long before we became family, so we had quite a history together. The phone rang just after 7 am, not a time when people usually call me, so I suspected a problem. It was my brother-in-law saying he thought that Polly had had a stroke. I could hear her making unintelligible noises, so I suspected he was right. We live close to town, and we were in the ER waiting for the ambulance to arrive. Michael was pacing, and I was just waiting to see Polly. I knew that when

9

Brain Attack

I saw her, I would know on some level how bad things were.

Eric walked though the door looking stunned but saying, "She's fine." Polly was sitting on the stretcher looking incredibly alert. As soon as she saw me, she extended one of her hands to me. When I looked into her eyes, I knew the Polly I loved was in there. Relief flooded through me. I squeezed her hand and told her I would see her in a minute. Eric told us the details of the attack. He knew exactly when it had occurred, which would be crucial information. The nurses and ER doctor made their assessment quickly, and the doctor came out to talk with the three of us.

The doctor's initial impression was that she had suffered a stroke and would be admitted to the hospital. Michael and Eric were happy to have me do the talking, and I kept waiting for the rest of the doctor's plan of treatment. None was forthcoming. Although my professional background is in mother-child nursing, I knew about the drug tPA and its use in the immediate treatment of stroke and heart attacks. When I asked when Polly would receive tPA, the doctor seemed shocked and told me sternly that it was considered experimental and had dangerous side effects.

Even if I wasn't a surgical nurse, I knew that tPA was not considered experimental, so I pursued the issue. I told the doctor that Polly was a public speaker. Given her comparatively young age and general good health, the apparent location of the stroke in the speech center of her brain, and the fact that we knew exactly when she had the attack, she was an excellent candidate for the drug. I asked the doctor to consult a neurologist at the medical center about 40 miles away. He agreed to do that. As soon as the neurologist there heard the parameters of Polly's case, he said she needed a CAT scan to document the stroke and make sure she was suffering from a clot and not a hemorrhage. Then they could administer tPA.

While this was happening, the three of us had been at Polly's bedside. She remained incredibly alert. The nurses immediately understood Polly's need to have me with her because she was unable to speak. I knew that she would want to know everything that was happening. In order for her to understand what I said to her, I had to be right in front of her when I spoke. We found out later that she was reading my lips. When anyone spoke to her, she would look at me for explanation or confirmation.

Meanwhile, the clock was ticking, and no tPA had been given. The neurologist from Copley came, read the CAT scan, and supported the use of tPA. This drug, however, had been administered only once in the previous year at Copley, and the staff was nervous about giving it. The ER doctor warned Eric, Michael, and me that tPA had a "high" complication rate, primarily hemorrhage, and that some patients did not survive. When I asked how high, he answered seven percent. Some people might think that's a large risk, but it said to me that 93 percent of patients did well. While the odds seemed good to me, the decision was Polly's.

10

When I asked the doctors if they had talked to Polly about tPA, they answered, "No." I asked Eric, "Don't you think we need to talk to her about this?" So off to her bedside we went. I leaned over her bed so I could be as close to her face as possible and she would easily see my lips. I explained about the side effects of tPA including death and asked if she understood. She nodded her head. I asked if she wanted to get tPA, and she nodded her head vigorously. Eric and I told the doctors to go ahead. Throughout the discussion, Polly was clutching my hand as if drawing strength from me. She was trapped in every health-care professional's worst nightmare--having a serious illness in a hospital where you know no one.

Because of the drug's potential side effects, Polly had to be transferred to the hospital in Burlington. She would need to be in the neurology intensive care unit for at least one day after the infusion of the drug. It is important for tPA to be administered within three hours after the stroke, and I was getting increasingly nervous as the minutes ticked by. Patience is not my strong suit, and when Polly's CAT scan had to be repeated, I was ready to jump out of my skin. We were running out of time. I prayed for calm. Exactly three hours after Polly's stroke, the tPA intravenous infusion was begun. The administration of the drug would have to continue in the ambulance, which meant that if Polly had significant side effects during the ride, not much could be done. Polly understood this. When she was asked if she wanted Eric to ride with her in the ambulance, she shook her head and pointed to me.

Eric and Michael were still trying to understand the impact of what had happened to Polly. It would be weeks before we would know the full extent of her brain attack, but we were reassured by her ability to make decisions. Our Polly was there, just not talking, although she was trying to do that too.

The nursing staff in the ER in the medical center was calming, helpful, and reassuring. Polly had to urinate almost immediately after she arrived, and they offered her a bedpan. She would have none of that, so the nurse brought her a bedside commode. Small measures such as that can go far toward preserving an ill person's dignity and independence.

In a relatively short time, three neurology residents–the house staff–arrived. As soon as they started talking, I knew we were in trouble. All three spoke with heavy accents. After Polly reacted blankly to the chief resident's first questions, he looked at me. Polly and I were trying not to laugh. Here was a brain-injured woman who was struggling to understand and communicate in English, and she was being asked complicated questions in heavily accented English about what had happened to her. Her look to me was, "What are they thinking?" Surely these trained professionals should have known how to talk to aphasic patients. When they got nowhere with their approach, they simplified their questions. That quickly frustrated Polly. She wasn't retarded; she had aphasia. I hadn't had a stroke, but I could barely understand the doctors either. Polly was depending on me, and neither one of us could understand much.

Off to the ICU we went. The ER nurses must have told the ICU staff that Polly responded better with me around because it just was assumed that where she went I went too. They got me a cot so I could spend the night with her. Little could I imagine how much fun we would have, and how quickly she would develop skills to deal with her new limitations.

I didn't know how soon Polly would show improvement from the tPA. To determine if there was any change, I asked her questions about people or things familiar to both of us. I asked her how many children she had, and she held up three fingers. I asked her oldest son's name, and she said the usual "brank." I felt like laughing, but I didn't want to upset her. Then I asked her second son's name, and she said, "Prick." I couldn't help myself, and I burst out laughing. Polly wanted to know what was so funny. I asked her if she wanted to know what she had just called Mark. She nodded, I told her, and she laughed too. Finally, I asked her youngest son's name, and after a moment of thought, she said, "Sex." The stress of the day and fatigue took over, and I really laughed. When I told Polly what she had said to get that reaction from me, she roared. Here we were, in the middle of the night, laughing so loudly that the nurse had to check on us.

Every hour after Polly's admission, the nurse did a full neurological assessment. After the third or fourth exam, Polly had memorized the sequence of the evaluation and anticipated the responses the nurse was looking for. One of the night nurses figured this out, and when she changed the routine, Polly was caught in her act. That was the beginning of Polly's developing compensatory behaviors to cope with the losses from the stroke.

<u>Michael</u>

I was sleeping late, and my wife, Jane, awakened me by saying, "Get up. Your sister is having a stroke." I was stunned for a moment, taking in the words and what they meant. "We have to meet them at the hospital," she continued.

I was up instantly, "Are you sure?"

"Eric said she fell on the treadmill and can't talk. I could hear her in the background, and she was making no sense."

I was dressed in two minutes; we were in the car in five minutes and at the hospital in ten. I know little medicine, relying on my wife and sister to explain medical jargon to me. When Paulina came in on a gurney, she seemed fine, but she had a frightened look in her eyes. Then she said, "Brank." She said other words, but they were unintelligible. I went to her side. She took my hand and kissed it. My heart broke. My sister was always smarter than I. She skipped a grade in school and always made better grades than I could ever dream of. Yet there she was on a gurney speaking a language no one, not even she, understood.

Jane took charge and talked with the ER doctor and neurologist. She convinced them to administer tPA. The day before I didn't know what tPA was, but I was learning fast. If the drug caused uncontrolled bleeding en route to Burlington, Paulina could suffer further damage, even die. Although the chances of that happening were small, that is not what you want to hear someone saying about your only sister. Jane would accompany Paulina in the ambulance. I would take Eric home to get his car, then return home to get some things for Jane before meeting them at the hospital.

While I drove home, I called our parents in San Antonio, Texas, on the car phone. I tried to break the news to them gently. I told them that Paulina had had a stroke and was being taken to a larger hospital. I left out the danger of further bleeding or death. I couldn't bring myself to tell our parents that their only daughter was in peril when they were so far away. I promised I would keep them posted.

On arriving at the medical center, I was directed to the intensive care unit. I found that the move had been accomplished without incident. Paulina was talking but making no sense. You could tell she was comprehending what you said, but she was unable to respond with anything but a movement of her head. When she didn't understand, you had to repeat yourself. I found that I was raising my voice. It suddenly occurred to me that she wasn't deaf, just confused, and what a dope I was for shouting.

I spent the rest of the day in the hospital with Eric, Jane, and Paulina. I drove home after dark, again calling our parents on the car phone. I explained that time would tell if the drug would help the situation. They wanted to know what damage the stroke had done. I tried to remain calm as I explained that my smart sister, of whom I was always so proud, was speaking in a tongue that made no sense. But my emotions welled up. I pulled off the road and cried for my sister.

Brain Attack

Marje

I was in my office seeing patients when I got a call that I knew must be serious to warrant my being interrupted. I left for the emergency room immediately. When I got there, they told me that Polly was leaving right away for the larger hospital and I didn't have much time to talk to her.

Polly was surrounded by Jane, Michael, and Eric. Jane looked as if she was in control. Michael wore an expression of disbelief. Eric seemed not to have grasped the situation yet. Polly looked frightened. She held my hand and asked in a very limited way, "Will I be all right?" It seemed to me that Polly was as fearful of going to another hospital as of the stroke itself. I kept telling Polly that she would be okay and that I would see her later in Burlington. That seemed to reassure her because she knew that she would have another advocate in that large health-care system.

That night in Burlington, I felt that the ICU staff was very understanding of Polly's emotional and physical needs. When the resident came in to ask Polly questions, however, I realized right away that Polly couldn't hear what he was saying and she was reading his lips. He seemed to ignore her hearing loss, as it didn't fit the usual stroke pattern.

Bryan

I wrote an e-mail to my mom telling her that I knew she would pull through okay. She and I have the same genes, and we are very determined, and she reminded me of that every day as I was growing up. I told her that I loved her and we would get through this together. I reminded my mom that when I finished law school and graduate school, I wasn't planning to go to school anymore. I kidded her that she was going to make me break my promise because I would have to go to school to learn sign language.

Scott

I received a phone call from a relative who told me that my mother had suffered a stroke and was in the hospital. It was such devastating news that I wanted to deny it, but knew that I couldn't. Having worked as an emergency medical technician for two years, I know what a stroke can do to a person. One second you're a whole person, and the next second you're an invalid who has to be taken care of.

As the hours went by, I felt helpless. There was my mother, with whom I have always had a very special relationship, in a hospital thousands of miles away. This was going to be the hardest thing for me to deal with for the next few months. I wanted to fly out to Vermont to see her and to assure her that

I loved her and would do everything in my power to make sure she had the best care in the hospital. Unfortunately, I was in no financial situation to afford the plane fare, and I was starting paramedic school in a few weeks. So I was left with having to listen to my mother make unintelligible sounds on the phone and with hoping that she understood what I was telling her. My father and my older brother were with her, but that did nothing to console me.

I hated the feeling of helplessness. No matter how bad a call I ever got on my ambulance, I could always do something to feel that I was making a difference, but now I could do nothing, and it was tearing me apart.

What Next ?

December 10, 1998

Life shrinks or expands in proportion to one's courage.

Anais Nin

I received a beautiful flower arrangement from my son Mark and his girl-friend Jamie. I was glad that the hospital didn't have the silly rule about no flowers in the ICU. I love flowers, and they reminded me that Mark and Jamie loved me.

It seemed that I was in a long, dark tunnel where the stroke had sucked out part of my life.

I tried to focus on a goal–speaking again–even though I felt as if a bomb had dropped into my life. I had never thought what it would mean to have words inside me and no way to share them with those around me, who for the moment could only guess at my feelings and needs. A speech therapist came in, gave Eric five strategies to help him communicate with me, and then told him that she was going on vacation and someone else would work with me. The strategies Eric learned were 1) write down short, simple sentences; 2) pantomime things he wanted me to do; 3) encourage me to use gestures; 4) give me specific feedback, and 5) take breaks and use key words.

I felt like a tiny boat, battered by a storm-tossed sea. I felt detached, floating on the sea. On that first day at the medical center, people talked at me, not to me. I nodded a lot because I couldn't speak, but I wanted to tell people things. I wanted them to see that I understood what they said. I wanted for everyone to hold my hand to ground me because I felt that my life was in shambles and the boat was in danger of capsizing. I knew that I was not in charge of much, and I felt helpless but not hopeless. Being in peril had sharpened my sense of life.

I wanted to shut out the frenzy and commotion around me. My mind wandered, and I couldn't pay attention when peopled talked to me. The constant flurry of hospital personnel overwhelmed me.

Doctors came in and asked me if I knew what month it was. I couldn't tell them, not because I didn't know but because I couldn't talk. I frantically gestured toward a calendar on the wall. The doctors didn't understand what I wanted, but Jane did, and she took the calendar down from the wall and gave it to me. Then I answered their question by pointing to December. What would have happened to me if Jane wasn't there? I suppose they would have thought I was no better.

I knew that they were trying to measure my cognitive impairment. They were doing a mini mental–state examination like the following:

MENTAL-STATE EXAMINATION

ORIENTATION

What is the (year) (season) (day) (month)?

Where are we: (state) (county) (town) (hospital) (floor)?

REGISTRATION

Name three unrelated objects. Allow one second to say each. Ask the patient to repeat all three after you have said them. Give one point for each correct answer. Repeat them until he or she learns all three.

ATTENTION AND CALCULATION

Ask patient to count backwards from 100 by seven. Give one point for each correct answer. Stop after five numbers.

RECALL

Ask patient to recall the three objects previously stated. Give one point for each correct answer.

LANGUAGE

Show patient a wristwatch; then ask patient what it is. Repeat for a pencil.

Ask patient to repeat the following: "No ifs, ands, or buts."

Ask patient to follow a three-stage command: "Take a paper in your right hand, fold it in half, and put it on the floor."

Ask patient to read and obey the following sentence that you have written on a piece of paper: "Close your eyes."

Ask patient to write a sentence.

Ask patient to copy a design.

I never thought much about the direction of my life; I was too busy living it. But the stroke jolted me into composing a mission statement for my life. On the first days I thought to myself, "I will be better." I knew that I was in charge of my health, and it was up to me to change illness into strength. I felt that I could handle whatever life had dished out. I wasn't able to ask for the menu, but I would do the best that I could.

Even though my mind was muddled, I decided that I could do three things: give up, fight, or change. My coping style allowed only two of those. Giving up was not an option to me, so I knew that I would fight, change, and heal. I would need others to support me, love me, and teach me the things I needed to learn. I knew that I had formidable challenges ahead.

My vocabulary had been whittled to a few misspoken words. I needed to find the vital missing link in my mind so that I could speak again. When I started trying to deal with the aphasia that accompanied the stroke, I felt the way I did when I took a vacation in Germany. I can't speak German. The Germans couldn't understand me, and I couldn't understand them. My German friends who spoke English had to translate everything for me. Not being able to talk felt the same way. The barrage of words people said made little sense to me.

I still couldn't hear very well, and the sounds that I could hear seemed to be muffled. I read facial expressions and people's lips even though I didn't know I could do that. I was not totally helpless, but the reality of not being able to speak was slowly sinking in.

MEDICAL FACTS

The days that follow the stroke are filled with diagnostic tests and usually by evaluations by a multi-disciplinary team of speech, occupational, and physical therapists to facilitate recovery.

drKoop.com

My mood plunged when I was moved from the ICU to a regular room, and the nurses told me that Jane couldn't stay with me at night. I panicked immediately. I felt like a rag blowing in the wind. The nurses kept telling me that no one could stay with me, and I kept gesturing, "No." I knew that I needed my family around me, but I couldn't make the nurses understand how I felt. As usual, Jane understood me. She negotiated. She asked the nurses if she could sit in a chair by my bed all night. The nurses agreed, provided the other patient in my room didn't mind. So Jane would spend the night sleeping in an uncomfortable chair so that I could feel safe. I couldn't understand why the nurses didn't see that I needed someone with me. I thought they would appreciate having someone to help them and me, but that was not the case. I wanted those nurses to be like the nurses in the ICU–caring and compassionate people who understood what I needed.

Jane went home to rest during the day. When my friend Marje arrived, she found me trying to get out of bed. I had intravenous lines (IVs) in place, and the bed's side rails were up, but I was already half way out of the bed. I was trying to get to the bathroom. I had rung my buzzer numerous times, but no one had answered. Being a nurse, Marje quickly helped me out of bed and into the bathroom. The buzzer was ringing and flashing the whole time. The nurse came in after I was back in bed. She told Marje that she had to make me realize that the nurses were very busy and would answer my buzzer when they could. Marje looked aghast when the nurse said that to her. That was not the kind of care that she and I gave our patients, and the comment shocked both of us.

Marje told me that several nurses had been sitting around at the nurses' station, chatting away and ignoring my buzzer. They kept shutting it off. I couldn't believe that the nurses were so cavalier about my needs.

To help me, Marje put a sign on my wall that said that everyone should speak slowly when taking to me. She also put up a sign for me to see that said "patience." Patience is not my strongest suit.

She asked if I knew lip reading. When I shook my head no, she told me that it seemed that I was watching people speak. She thought that I did have some knowledge of lip reading. That night I thought I could hear better. Marje reassured me that even though my words and thoughts weren't connecting right, I was getting better.

My son Scott, who was an emergency medical technician, called, but I couldn't hear him on the phone. Marje took the phone and wrote me a message from Scott telling me that he loved me and was worried about me and to hang tough.

Michael wrote me a note that he had a surprise for me.

Jane

I began to feel real dread for what might lie ahead for Polly. In the day since the tPA was given, I hadn't seen much improvement. I wanted results fast. Maybe the drug wasn't going to work, but what else could we have done?

After the ICU, everything about Polly's care became a struggle. She required little in the way of direct nursing care beyond monitoring her IV. Eric, Marje, and I, together and separately, tried to forge a bond with the nursing staff. We wanted to become a team with them to maximize Polly's treatments. Instead, the nursing staff saw us as the enemy and took it out on Polly.

None of us knew how to begin speech and occupational therapy, but we all knew that after a stroke rehabilitation needs to begin quickly. At last the residents ordered therapists to come and evaluate Polly.

Brain Attack

Marje

Polly's transfer to her room was most upsetting to me. After I helped her to the bathroom and put her back in bed, I asked her if she had rung for the nurse, and she replied, "A lot." When the nurse finally came in, she said, "You will have to tell this patient to just be patient and wait. I am very busy, and there are many other people whose needs have to be met."

The lab technician who came to draw Polly's blood was kind and patient and seemed to be more understanding. She had a conversation with Polly about giving birth with midwives. She was actually interested in Polly as a person.

Polly struggled with trying to get her thoughts across to all of us. It didn't take us long to realize that even though Polly couldn't talk, she understood what we were saying. We discovered that if we wrote down what we were saying, we could communicate with her very well, but it took time and patience to help Polly get her thoughts across.

December 11, 1998

***Don't think there are no crocodiles
because the water is calm.***

A Malayan Proverb

The crisis was over, but the damage would continue for a long time. I couldn't tell anyone how I felt, as I was almost mute. My nearly wordless life was like a barren landscape. Time was measured not in hours and minutes, but by the time it took me to say one word.

I felt that the brain attack had stolen my identity. I was on center stage of a play that was my life. The cast of characters changed continuously as people moved into and out of my room. I had to decide what part I had in this play as the rest of the cast revolved around me. I guessed that I must be playing the lead. That confused me as I couldn't even lead myself.

I didn't seem to have the ability to organize my thoughts very well, and everything seemed topsy-turvy and askew. I couldn't follow a conversation. I tried to register the meaning of the words that people were saying but to no avail. The effort to think was huge. I was tired.

I am an intelligent, well-educated woman and I hated it when health-care professionals talked down to me, as if I were a child. Jane helped me with that. She wouldn't let people dismiss me or my need to know what was happening to me.

My brother brought me an e-mail message from my mother and dad that said they were thinking about me all the time. They said that many people in their neighborhood were saying prayers for me. They told me not to get discouraged and to grit my teeth and keep trying.

My mind was still awash with confusion, and my head felt queer. What was going on in my brain? I felt as if I was lost in a crowd, but there was no crowd.

Jane tried to help me start recuperating, even though I was profoundly confused most of the time. No one at the hospital was telling us much, so Jane started teaching me herself. She played tic tac toe with me. I couldn't write, but I could make the X's. I won some of the games too. Jane also asked me to try to write, "Hang tough!" I couldn't write it with my right hand very well, but I could do it with my left hand even though I'm not left-handed. I kept wondering when the speech therapist would come.

As is usual in a teaching hospital, residents provided most of the medical care. The attending doctor breezed in once in a while. Most of the communication came in the form of explanations by the junior neurology resident. He realized that I needed more explanations than the average patient, and he took the time to draw diagrams and help me understand what tests he was ordering. I still had trouble hearing, so Eric wrote much of what was said to me. I could read what he wrote just fine.

The process of saying a word confused me. What did I do first? I couldn't say many words, and the ones that I could say were strange and fractured. It seemed that the stroke had locked up my words in a prison.

Here in the medical center none of the doctors seemed to be interested about my psyche–how I felt inside. Many doctors don't seem to know anything about the soul. I wondered if they realized that I had a psyche or a soul.

I was scheduled for a test, and I asked several times if Jane would be able to go with me. The resident always answered yes. When I got to the room for the transesophageal echocardiogram (which looks for abnormalities in the heart that might have contributed to the stroke), I was sedated, and Jane was told to leave. Even though I was heavily sedated, I knew that Jane was not there, and I started fighting the attendants. They gave me even more sedative and decided that I would do better if Jane was there. They allowed her back into the room, but the damage was done. Even though the test only took 15 minutes, the ill effects lasted much longer. Because I had been over-medicated, I slept all day and most of the night and had nothing to eat all day.

Sleeping all day, I didn't know that Michael had brought me a surprise,

Brain Attack

which was that my son Bryan had flown from Dallas to see me. I didn't see him until the next day. When I awakened, I felt tricked. I couldn't trust the doctors anymore. They had robbed me of knowing my son was there. Their betrayal exacerbated the trauma of the stroke.

Jane

Where were the therapists? Every time I asked what the hold-up was, I was told someone was checking. A speech therapist had seen Polly only once--for a few minutes when Polly was admitted to the hospital.

Eric

Our son was upset with me when, after two days, I asked Polly to tell me how to get our e-mails off the computer. He thought it was too soon for her to do that, but after being married to this woman for 35 years I knew that she had the answer. If my asking bothered her, she would let me know. Sure enough, she was able to tell me how to do it even though she couldn't speak. At that point I knew she would be okay. I knew that if she kept her mind working, she would eventually overcome her other problems.

Bryan

Before I got to the hospital, people kept trying to brace me for how my mother looked. When I saw her, she looked okay to me, maybe a little weak, but nothing to panic about. She seemed really happy to see me. By looking in my mother's eyes, I knew that she would be okay. I couldn't understand what people were talking about. I guess they didn't have the bond with my mother that I did.

Some people were talking to her as if she was retarded. God that pissed me off! Couldn't they see it wasn't the incoming information but the outgoing information that was messed up? I tried to act not quite as if nothing was wrong but certainly not as if she was an idiot. I figured a little intellectual respect would make her feel better. It seemed stupid to do otherwise.

Mother's stroke kind of blew my dad away, and he said to me, "That was supposed to have been me in this bed, not your mother." He seemed real serious and nervous, so I spent time with him trying to make him understand that it would be okay, then and in the future. I am like my mother in some respects, and we don't freak out in situations like that. We just execute.

Some of the things she tried to say were comical, even to her. She kept trying to say my brothers' names, and she said, "Prick" and "Sex." She laughed and laughed because she knew those weren't their names, and she didn't know why she called them that. I knew she would be all right if she could laugh at herself.

22

Scott

After a few days, my mother was able to say a word or two. On the telephone I told her that I loved her and wanted to be with her. She listened quietly. I asked if she understood me, and she said one word, "Yes." That simple word made me feel so much better.

I was concerned about mother's mental capacity. She had always been available to give me advice and make me feel better when I was frustrated with life, so I was crushed to think that the relationship we shared might never be the same. This fear eased as the days went by. I would ask my father and brother if she was the same inside as she had been. They assured me she was. I didn't believe them until one day when I was calling I heard my mother trying to explain to my father the process of retrieving her e-mail. I thought that if she could tell him how to accomplish that just a couple days after a stroke, there was no limit to what was ahead.

December 12, 1998

Injustice anywhere is a threat to justice everywhere.
Dr. Martin Luther King, Jr.,
Letter from a Birmingham Jail
April 16, 1963

When I awoke, Bryan was there. His trip across the country made me realize that I had done a good job of raising him and that I was important to him. Seeing him gave me a feeling of peace. Being able to hold his hand meant a lot to me.

When the neurology resident examined me in the morning, I couldn't understand what he was saying. Eric wrote down the doctor's questions. Even the most basic information baffled me, and I depended on Eric and Jane to interpret for me.

The turmoil continued. I thought that I would be all right by myself, so I told Jane that she could go home to sleep. Was I wrong! A headache claimed me. My neck and shoulders were riddled with tension, and when my family went home, I was sleeping in a reclining chair to ease my neck. Later I decided that I might be able to sleep in the bed. At about 3 am, a

Brain Attack

nurse came into my room and appeared to be removing my recliner. In my rudimentary language, I pleaded with her not to take the chair away because I might need to rest in it again that night. I gesticulated frantically to make myself understood. I managed to say, "Please, no." It was to no avail. The nurse said in a loud, forceful voice, "No. You just watch me." Her arms were locked around her chest. She was telling me in actions, not words, that she was in control. For a moment, I thought she was so angry, she would hit me.

The nurse shoved the chair out of the room and pushed it down the hallway just enough that I could see it but couldn't get it. I felt like a dog in a cage, and I wanted Bryan and Eric to come so I could get out. The nurse's display of power and indifference astounded me. Why should she be so vindictive? I could see her face in my mind even after she left the room. It seemed to have written on it the words "brute authority." You never believe that something like this is going to happen to you. My innocence and my trust were violated, and I felt hysteria welling up in my throat. With sheer will, I made myself go back to sleep.

I thought the abuse was over, but at about 5 am I awoke needing to go to the bathroom. Because my whole right side was weakened from the stroke, I couldn't go by myself. I rang my buzzer for the nurse. A different nurse came in, and in my language of gestures, I asked her for help. She asked me what my name was. My name was on my arm band, but I couldn't say it. I gestured at my arm band and slipped it around my wrist so she could see it better. She asked me my name again, but I couldn't tell her. I couldn't say the word Polly. Four times I tried to talk to ask her for help. She seemed to be purposely toying with me. By then I needed the bathroom badly. At last she said, "Okay, I'll let you go," and she laughed. My soul felt ripped in a thousand pieces. I was humiliated. I was scared. I felt completely alone.

I was being treated like an inconvenience and a bother to the nurses instead of like a patient they should care for. Where were their feelings? Did they know there was a human being inside my skin? I couldn't fathom why they were in nursing if they didn't want to take care of patients. Even though I had been in the health-care field for 35 years, I must have been naive not to think that nurses could be so spiteful. I knew that nurses are overworked and pressured by changes in the health-care system, but that didn't excuse their inhumanity. I was ashamed to be a nurse.

December 13, 1998

It is an equal failing to trust everybody and to trust nobody.

18th century proverb.

What more could they do to me? I didn't want to know, so I didn't ask for help for the rest of the night. I lay awake fighting panic until I thought the nursing shifts had changed. My head was throbbing with exhaustion. I subdued the panic inside me by visualizing that everything was all right and that Eric would get me out of there. I told myself that crying would upset me more and that I had to wait until someone in my family could get me out of the mess that was called nursing care. I lay in the dark and tried to rehearse in my head the words I would say to Eric and Bryan when they arrived. I needed to get out of that hospital

They came at about 7:30 am. In my elementary speech, I pleaded with them to get me out of there. I managed to speak. The first full sentence I spoke after the brain attack was, "Get me out of here."

The pain in my adult son's eyes when he knew that his mother had been frightfully abused will be in my mind forever. He kept telling me that he and his father would fix it. I didn't want them to fix it. I just wanted to be out of this hospital.

With the help of a nurse friend and the neurologist at Copley, I left that afternoon and was transferred back to Copley, the hospital where I had started. The incident had an earth-shaking impact on me. I wondered if the neurologist at Copley had given Eric her home phone number because she knew that I might need to get out of the teaching hospital. When the medical center doctor discharged me, it was in the manner of a monologue with directives telling me that I'd be back for rehab. A tide of anger rose inside me. I knew that I would never go back there. My level of trust in that hospital was irreversibly broken. Why would I want to go back to a place where I had been abused? I had had a stroke, but I hadn't lost my mind.

The week was a downward spiral into chaos–the violent brain attack, being unable to communicate with words, and being traumatized in the hospital. There was a sense of relief in admitting that everything was out of control. In the ambulance on the trip to Copley, I let out emotions that I had kept in check all day. My emotions reigned.

Brain Attack

Eric

When I entered Polly's hospital room in the morning, she was sitting on the bed sobbing, and she said to me, "Get me out of here." This was the first whole sentence I had heard her say since the stroke.

Our good nurse friend and the neurologist at Copley came to my rescue when they arranged for Polly to transfer out of the medical center hospital.

Marje

I was paged in church in the morning. It was Eric telling me that Polly was going to sign herself out of the hospital in Burlington. I called the neurologist, Dr. Prunty, who agreed to take Polly as a transfer patient. I then talked to one of the neurology residents, who kept telling me that they couldn't transfer a patient on Sunday. I told him that if necessary I would talk to the CEO at Copley and have her call the medical center hospital to expedite Polly's transfer. I called Eric again and told him that if we couldn't get Polly to Copley on Sunday, I would go to Burlington and stay with her until Monday morning.

Jane

We were told that Polly needed to stay at the medical center hospital because they could offer her more rehabilitative services than our local hospital. We took them at their word--a decision we all later regretted. In retrospect, we should have been more assertive, but we didn't want to rock the boat, and as a result nothing substantive happened. And it was not just we who were ignored. The attending neurologist at the medical center hospital wouldn't return phone calls from the referring neurologist from our local hospital. Thank heaven the referring neurologist gave Eric and me her home phone number because she answered many questions for us and helped us get Polly admitted to Copley after the nighttime fiasco. The night nurses belittled, humiliated, and emotionally traumatized Polly so badly that I worried that she would be scarred forever. For a medical professional to treat an aphasic patient the way Polly was treated is akin to beating her. In retrospect, it was a bad decision on our part to let her stay by herself at night. Because of the nursing staff's resistance to my staying with Polly at night, I had convinced her that she was better and stronger and that the nurses would care for her. Polly reluctantly agreed to stay alone because I was tired and because Eric and Bryan would stay with her until she went to sleep.

Chapter Two
I Can Spot Excellence Quickly

*The future belongs to those who believe in the
beauty of their dreams.*

Eleanor Roosevelt

Coming to Copley restored my dignity. In that small rural hospital, I began to rebuild my life. When I came in, the first nurse I had seen in the ER after the stroke stopped what she was doing and waved hello. I knew then that everything was going to be all right. The nurse never knew what her gesture meant to me and how she helped erase my feeling that nurses were the enemy. Health care is about the relationship between the healer and the patient, but in health care these days there's too little time for communicating. Copley, however, had a reputation for tender, loving care, which I desperately needed. The staff had been told about my mistreatment, and they worked to earn my trust. In their kind words and gestures, they conveyed respect for me. I didn't feel that Jane needed to be my shield or that my family had to stay at night. I saw that the nurses remembered what the phrase "health professional" meant, and they had no need to assert their control over patients.

MEDICAL FACTS

Nurses work on several levels--physical, medical, emotional, and nurturing--and interact with the patient's family and friends. The nurse has the most frequent and closest contact with the hospitalized patient.

I knew that I couldn't control what came next, so I decided to use what had happened to my benefit. The dance of life had continued for me, but I was uncertain what step to make next. I had to learn new choreography. I had to trust that the brain attack had carried me to the place I most needed to be at that time in my life.

FROM THE NEUROLOGIST

On a Sunday morning four days after I initially saw Polly, her husband called to say that Polly wanted to leave the medical center hospital. I agreed to make the arrangements for her transfer back to Copley. I was glad that Polly would be in my care again.

I was happily amused with her persistence and insistence about getting optimal care and attention. Quickly I noticed how she pushed herself and everyone around her to give their best. She would accept nothing less. It was clear that as a physician I would be working with her, not on her.

I admired her drive and feisty spirit, as I knew that pluck and resilience would be the most important determinants in her recovery. The brain attack had faced a serious challenger in Polly. She refused to give up or give in.

Jane

The transfer occurred late in the afternoon, and all of us breathed a sigh of relief when Polly was wheeled into Copley. When I asked her if she wanted me to stay with her, she shook her head no and said, "Don't need." She felt safe, and we did too.

Marje

I called the head of the physical therapy (PT) department at Copley to see if they would be able to meet Polly's rehabilitation needs. Contrary to what I had been told at Burlington, the head of the PT department assured me that Polly would have good comprehensive therapy at Copley.

Maureen

I spoke to Polly for the first time after her stroke. Her speech was very slow, and it was painful to hear her. I wanted to talk for her so that she wouldn't have to work so hard.

December 14, 1998

Two are better than one
For if they fall, one will lift up his fellow.

Ecclesiastes 4:9-10

I felt safe, ensconced in a secure place. On my second day in Copley, I faced reality when I met Donna, the woman who would be my speech therapist. The sooner that speech therapy begins, the more effective it is likely to be so Donna went to work quickly. I was nervous and tense from my head to my feet, but I was not daunted by the task in front of me. I had to be able to talk again

---

MEDICAL FACTS

Speech and language pathologists identify loss of motor or language function and communication skills. They also evaluate swallowing function. They work with those who have aphasia as the result of a stroke.

It's so silent when you can't talk. I was still dazed and confused. The way I experienced the world had changed. I was on a voyage of discovery. I both feared and welcomed the future.

Five days had passed since my stroke. I knew that for the time being Donna knew more about speaking than I did. But asking her for help frightened me. What if she mistreated me too? I learned the answer quickly. In our first meeting, Donna said something that endeared her to me. I know she talked about a lot of things, but the only thing that I remember was that she said she would always be honest with me. Honesty is very important to me. I have always told my clients that they could depend on me to say the truth, so I thought that the client/therapist relationship with Donna was off to a good start.

Donna wrote her name on a piece of paper, but I kept forgetting it. Sometimes I had a distant flash of memory about her name, but usually she had to repeat it. She asked me to say her name, but I couldn't. I tried valiantly, but nothing came out. I was awash with confusion.

It's heady stuff starting over like a newborn baby, but if I could start from the beginning once, I could do it again. Since I did well with my first experience in speaking, I could speak again. I just had to learn how.

I could read, but letters on a page held no meaning unless I saw them as a whole word.

The catalog of aphasia terms that described what happened to me was a long one. The huge terms and their definitions made me feel that I was stranded in treacherous waters. Before the stroke, a word was nothing I ever thought about. After the stroke, I found that a word was a memorized link between a sound and a meaning. I had to learn to connect the sound with the idea of a word again. It seemed so hard to me.

Speech therapy is methodical and step by step, and I was at the beginning of the learning curve. I had to find a way to use my remaining skills and learn compensatory techniques of communication. I told myself that I was alive and I could do anything that I had to.

FROM THE SPEECH PATHOLOGIST

When I first met Polly Perez, it was in response to an evaluation request for a "young woman who had recently had a CVA [cerebrovascular accident]." She had just been transferred here from a hospital in a larger city. This transfer didn't make much sense, as it would usually have been in the opposite direction. A person with a CVA might initially be admitted to the tiny local hospital but would then be transferred to the larger city or regional hospital for extensive rehabilitation and outpatient treatment.

I entered the hospital room to see a petite woman whom I judged to be in her forties and a tall blonde woman who introduced herself as Polly's sister-in-law, Jane. Polly was sitting on the bed and quickly responded to my greetings with a smile and "Hi." Jane said, "Polly knows what she wants to say, but the words aren't coming out."

Polly had a very long list of communication disorders that included--in the technical terms speech therapists use--aphasia (receptive and expressive), cortical word deafness, anomia, alexia, surface and deep dyslexia, agraphia, acalculia, and apraxia.

Aphasia is a general term for a disorder of communication. Aphasia can be very mild and hardly noticeable or so severe that a person cannot speak or understand language and cannot read or recognize letters and numbers.

At the time of her stroke, Polly was at the severe end of the continuum. She had a few words in her vocabulary, but they were often garbled, and her speech was ungrammatical (agrammatism). She experienced great difficulty naming common items (anomia). In addition, she didn't understand much of what was being said to her (cortical deafness). She could read some words, but individual letters of the alphabet made no sense to her when she looked at them or heard them spoken. She couldn't hear the differences in vowel sounds in such words as pat, pet, pit, and pot. The sounds and the symbols meant nothing to her. That is very much like a youngster who experiences dyslexia when learning to read and write. In addition, Polly couldn't write letters very well (agraphia). She couldn't spell words, and telling time was a struggle. She didn't recognize numbers or know basic arithmetic facts like multiplication or subtraction (acalculia). Money concepts also had to be relearned.

Polly also had great difficulty with motor planning, which is related to apraxia, often the most debilitating element of a brain attack. Injury to nerve pathways prevented Polly from saying the words she could form in her brain. As a result she knew what she wanted to say, but she couldn't get the words out right--either no words or mixed-up words. She often had to talk around a topic to make her needs known. Many people with apraxia not only do no not recover any functional speech, but they also are often unable to say more that a few automatic phrases, thus breaking the speaking and communication cycle forever.

With the results of a bedside evaluation complete, I realized that Polly had suffered from a severe and momentarily debilitating stroke. As I soon found out, Polly had had a long career as an internationally renowned public speaker about childbirth and maternity nursing. She had also written a number of highly regarded books in her field. Language had been central to her life for many years. What could the future hold for her? I could not consider alternatives other than recovery. As a therapist my role was to provide direct speech-therapy services to this woman. But where to start?

A look at things to come

Everything I will learn begins in rehab. Rehabilitation is not "one size fits all." A team of occupational, physical, and speech therapists developed the plan and goals for my rehabilitation. Those three people would support me until I could do things on my own. Their first goal was to create a secure, dynamic environment that inspired independence. The task before me was formidable, and I knew that I had to dig deep inside myself to find strength. I had always been a fierce competitor, and this challenge was not insurmountable. I would do it at full tilt.

MEDICAL FACTS

Rehabilitation often involves many professionals--physician, nurse, physical therapist, occupational therapist, speech and language therapist, psychologist, social worker, and chaplain--and the patient and her family and friends.

The major goal of stroke rehabilitation is to maximize the independence, lifestyle, and dignity of the patient and the family unit. No one person can be an expert in all of the areas listed, so there is a need for teamwork with the client and the family.

Rehabilitation aims at increasing the stroke survivor's independence, including: activities of daily living, mobility skills, communication skills, cognitive skills, socialization skills, and psychological health.

The family plays an important role in providing support and care and making decisions. The final decisions must remain with the patient and family.

Next, I met my occupational therapist, a vivacious young woman named Debbie. She started me on exercises that would help my right hand and arm. They seemed like they weren't mine, but I kept using them anyway. I started with dexterity- and manipulation- skills training. Debbie taught me how to place my palm flat on the bedside table, raising and lowering my fingers one by one. She told me that using my hand to do needlework would help too, so she gave me a small piece of needlepoint to do. Debbie's assignment was also to reteach me a multitude of tasks of daily living and skills such as math.

MEDICAL FACTS

The goal of occupational therapy (OT) is to restore a person's ability to perform activities of daily living. After an evaluation of the patient's perceptual and cognitive functions, the therapist works at stimulating and re-educating those functions. Often occupational therapists concentrate on retraining the upper extremities.

FROM THE OCCUPATIONAL THERAPIST

I was aware of the poor treatment Polly had received at the previous hospital, and I wondered whether she would be able to trust our therapy staff and nursing team. I realized that we had to earn her trust.

When I entered her room to introduce myself, Polly was reading a magazine. I immediately realized the severity of her speech difficulties. I tried to speak slowly with simple phases to give her time to process what I was saying, but at the same time I didn't want to insult her intelligence. I thought to myself how frustrating it must be to know the words in her mind but be unable to speak them. I knew from the patient chart that Polly had had a successful career as a public speaker, educator, and advocate for women. She tried to participate in the OT evaluation, and I admired her determination.

The evaluation showed that she had several deficits including poor fine motor coordination in her right hand, poor sensation in that hand, and poor hand control. These things would affect her ability to care for herself and do the many tasks she had done so easily at home and at work.

The first thing she communicated to me was a desire to regain the use of her hand, so that was where I started working. I gave her a sheet of exercises, theraputty to squeeze to strengthen her right hand, and a simple needlepoint/weaving activity to help her regain gross and fine motor control.

I began physical therapy as well. I had to learn exercises to strengthen my right leg and improve my balance. My first physical therapist was a woman named Carrie. She asked me to walk down the hall, and I knew she was observing my gait and stability. Since I have stairs in my home, she took me to the PT department and asked me to walk up and down two or three stairs. Then we progressed to walking up and down the stairs in the hospital.

I soon found myself mired in work. I started copying the letters of the alphabet so that my handwriting would improve, and I started trying to make the sounds of letters so I could eventually make words. The slightest effort, either mental or physical, depleted my total reserves, while the episodes in Burlington were still vivid in my mind.

Marje brought me some Christmas cookies on her way to work. That was such a thoughtful gesture. When she was here, I wanted to say the word "snow" so badly. I could see the fluffy, fleecy stuff through the window. I wanted to have that swift, sharp shock you get when you remember something you've been searching for. I tried to recall the word that described snow, but I couldn't recall anything. It took a lot of time for Marje to guess what word I wanted her to say so I could try to repeat it.

Michael and Jane brought me a Christmas cactus in the morning, and that gave me a little lift.

Brain Attack

Stephanie

When I called Polly, I wasn't sure what to expect. Polly had been at my home a few months before her stroke, just a couple of months before I found out that I was pregnant. As her phone rang, I wondered if she would remember me. What had happened to the mind I admired? What would happen to all of the knowledge that I wanted so much to take from her?

To my surprise, she seemed to recognize my name immediately. Even though she was having difficulty speaking, she asked about the baby I was expecting.

We spoke briefly. It was...awkward. The woman with the brilliant mind, my idol, was having difficulty forming simple sentences. It was painful to speak to her. It's difficult hearing someone you look up to strug-gling with her future and the unknown.

I got off the telephone and cried. I cried because of fear. Would my hero die? I cried about the unknown. Polly was alive, but would she ever be "Polly" again?

December 15, 1998

To hear the whispered voice of another's heart
and understand unspoken words
are the talents of those lucky few
people who are precious to the world.

Theresa Ann Hunt

I took stock of my condition. I knew that I couldn't talk and couldn't even connect the sequence of letters with the sequence of their sounds. I couldn't identify individual sounds within words. I thought to myself, "This is bad, really bad."

I was amazed that Donna and Debbie came back. They kept their word. In Burlington people said they would come back the next day, but no one did. I'll never forget how it felt when I knew that Donna had kept her promise to return. It was the beginning of a fragile trust between client and therapist.

Donna helped me form sounds in my mouth. It seemed easier to make the sounds when I saw her mouth work. Saying a word was excruciatingly slow. When you move so slowly through trying to say words, talking becomes a meditation. I had to open my mind and find where my words were stored. I knew they were in there somewhere. Donna has to help me uncover the words and phrases that are stashed away in my brain. She told me that in order to teach me to talk again she had to determine what I understood. She had to test my writing, reading, understanding of speech, and oral speech.

For the time being, I hated choices. It was too much to decide anything, so most of the time I just did what people asked. That was a decided change in my life.

The neurologist had told me that I should dress in "normal" clothes, so Eric brought me sweat pants and a sweatshirt. He picked out a sweatshirt that had a Christmas motif. I didn't feel "Christmasy" at all.

I didn't like having more than one person talk to me at one time. I wanted people to slow down when they spoke. What words I had seemed to be twisted around in my brain. Speaking felt unnatural and like an obstacle course. My thinking was mechanical and unfocused.

Although I once believed that words are vital for life, being almost wordless showed me that I could communicate without them. I was getting to be a master of gestures and pantomime. The lone word that I could occasionally say was like a solitary figure walking on a beach.

Donna told me that part of her job was to determine the amount of function I had lost and what passages for comprehension of language were available. She would assess the possibility that treatment might augment the function I still had. To test my auditory comprehension, Donna read me a list of numbers, such as 4, 8, 2, 6, and told me to state the largest one. We did only eight lists, but I did them all correctly.

I also said ten words correctly aloud (lamp, coat, radio, pen, window, salt, car, door, broom, eggs). When I said a word, I felt as if I was dawdling because it took forever to say anything.

Donna asked me to try to copy the movements that her mouth made when she said the words pot, pop, pom, pod, pat, pet, but I couldn't do it. It was a game of follow-the-leader that I couldn't follow,. I felt that I was wandering in the wilderness without words. Where were they?

One of my friends came to visit bearing a gift of flowers. Seeing the flowers cheered me up, as the scene I saw through my hospital window was rather arctic. I wanted desperately to say his name, but I couldn't. I knew who he was, his name had only three letters, but saying "Bob" was out of my reach.

I was alone with my thoughts, and I would retreat into my private, wordless world. When people spoke, I felt as if I was being bombarded by word missiles. My family, friends, and therapists became my translators.

Debbie gave me an ergonomic hand exerciser to strengthen my hand. It provided progressive resistance, and I used it several time times a day. She gave me clay to pull and form into balls to retrain the muscles in my hand. I used the clay whenever I was sitting in bed.

Debbie also taught me two upper-extremity coordination exercises. I was supposed to put my left hand on my left shoulder with my right arm stretched out in front at shoulder level and then bring my right hand to my right shoulder as I straightened out my left arm. I could do that exercise pretty well but not the next one. I had to place my hands on my knees, left palm up and right palm down, turn my hands over simultaneously so that my right palm was up and my left palm was down, and keep repeating it. I couldn't coordinate the movements.

I restrained myself from using my left arm so that I used my right arm more. I didn't want to coddle it.

The doctor who was to consult about my Coumadin therapy came to see me. Coumadin is a blood thinner that would prevent the formation of more clots like the one that had caused my stroke. There were no unoccupied chairs in my room, so after introducing himself, he sat down on the floor. This is a new way to do a consult, I thought. By sitting on the floor, he became more accessible to me. Smart man!

FROM THE SPEECH PATHOLOGIST

My first impression of Polly was of a determined woman who was eager to "get started" on the road to recovery and didn't want to waste one minute of the day or night. If I suggested that Polly should do something for an hour, she did it for five..I don't think she slept much while she was in the hospital. I knew from the nursing staff that she was up before dawn and stayed up late working on therapy tasks. She wasn't in the hospital to feel sorry for herself but to engage in therapy and soak it up like a sponge. Speech therapy, occupational therapy, and physical therapy--all of it.

FROM THE OCCUPATIONAL THERAPIST

When I came to Polly's room, I was amazed to find that she had finished the needlepoint I had given her the day before. She communicated that she was ready for a new set of exercises. She had mastered in one day the exercises that I gave her. Most patients would have needed two weeks. It was refreshing to meet someone so determined and so willing to take her recovery into her own hands.

MEDICAL FACT

Polly's instinct to force herself to use her right arm was validated by the results of a small study of stroke survivors in Germany and at the University of Alabama in Birmingham. In the study the good arm was immobilized while for several weeks the survivors had daily, intensive physical therapy on the disabled arm. The study showed that depending on the initial severity of their disability, stroke victims could recover up to 95 percent of the use of their arm. Brain imaging showed that the area of the brain that controlled the disabled limb increased during therapy, suggesting that new neural pathways had developed. The study was reported in the June 2000 issue of Stroke: Journal of the American Heart Association. Trials of the therapy were planned at the National Institutes of Health, in Bethesda, Maryland. The University of Alabama was also planning to use immobilization therapy to treat legs that had been disabled by a stroke.

Marje

So she would know her options, I talked to Polly about going to Dartmouth-Hitchcock Hospital in New Hampshire for extensive rehabilitation. She started crying and managed to convey that she feared she might be mistreated again. Polly felt safe at Copley and was afraid to go anywhere else. I felt sad that she had become so fragile in such a short time mainly because of her mistreatment in Burlington.

December 16, 1998

Freedom lies in being bold
Robert Frost

I wanted to take my bath before the day shift came on, as I had all my therapy to do, so I asked the nurse where the bathtub was. She asked me if I needed help, and I answered no. I wanted to bathe myself. As I saw it, I had to be able to do my daily living tasks myself. The bath took me a while, but I relished the independence of bathing myself. I bathed , put a towel on the floor, and sat on the towel to dress myself, so I wouldn't fall.

Thinking was harder than bathing. My thinking was slow and usually ineffectual. Ideas wouldn't come. I couldn't keep focused for very long when people talked. I felt like a remnant of who I used to be. I was desperate to hold on to my thoughts, but they kept floating away like clouds. It was easy to get confused, and most of the time I was physically and mentally exhausted. It seemed that I was combing through the shards of my life and couldn't make sense of the pieces.

I practiced saying Donna's name so that I could remember it and say it correctly. I worked on putting in the correct order the four steps needed to do a task, such as write a letter to a friend; put the letter into the envelope; put a stamp on the envelope; and mail the letter. I did them correctly.

When I saw something I knew, I couldn't say it, and sometimes I couldn't even describe it. It made me feel dumb even though I knew that I'm smart.

I was desperately trying to regain my footing in life. Michael brought his laptop computer to the hospital in the hope that it might help me communicate. I couldn't turn it on. It was confusing to me even though I knew what I needed to do with it.

I found a big bruise on my thigh from when I had the stroke and fell down trying to get off of the treadmill.

My room was filling with flowers, as I got several more bouquets . I get so much pleasure being surrounded by them. Not only are they beautiful but I seem to draw strength from them as I watch them go from bud to bloom. I hope that my speech will bloom too but right now it is still in a very tight bud.

My first attempts at writing looked like scribbling. I needed almost two inches just to write one letter of the alphabet. I sat in my hospital bed copying letters as I had done in grade school. The first words that I asked to be shown how to write were Eric, Jane, Marje, Bryan, Mike, Mark, and Scott. My stubborn nature helped a lot because I kept writing until I could do it better.

I was working on saying some words, and Donna gave me a set of cards with words on them. I tried to say some of the words, but my mind was like a computer gone awry because the words never got out of my mouth. The words in my mind lay dormant. I wondered if there was a parallel universe where my words had gone. Donna told me to watch her when I tried to say a word. In the beginning, when I heard language it sounded foreign to me like someone was speaking in Greek, not English.

Sometimes when I mispronounced a word, I was reminded of the saying, "This is good enough for government work," because the word wasn't right but it was good enough. No one knew that I wanted to say that phrase because I couldn't tell anyone.

I kept my right hand under a pillow at night so my fingers wouldn't curl up. During Debbie's visit, I asked in my rudimentary way how I could help my hand stay straight. I didn't like it when my hand looked crumpled. Debbie suggested that I work on picking up a pencil and rolling it between my thumb and fingers over and over again.

FROM THE SPEECH PATHOLOGIST

My first task as a therapist was to find Polly's strengths and to assist her in developing strategies to work with her weaknesses. Speaking was an obvious goal, but reading and writing were absolutely key to Polly's life and career. While the aphasia was severe, her cortical deafness meant that she knew that people were speaking to her, but the rhythm and sounds of speech were not connecting as words in her brain. In the first week, we worked through this deficit area so that she could understand what I was saying to her 75 percent of the time. Polly could recognize whole words in print, but she could not recognize individual letters of the alphabet nor hear those letters as recognizable sounds.

Pamela

I called Polly in the hospital. The call was short because she tired easily and she couldn't speak much. I was so upset to hear her garbled words. Here was a brilliant and powerful public speaker who couldn't speak. After the call, I cried and cried. I cried for all the people who might miss her ability to inspire them. I cried for those who needed her to motivate them to make changes in the health-care system. And I cried for Polly.

Brain Attack

December 17, 1998

The intent, and not the deed, is in our power,
and therefore who dares greatly does greatly.

Brown

I found my days were strange and filled with both exhaustion and determination.

I woke up early and practiced saying a whole sentence that I had in my mind. When a housekeeping lady came into the room, I pointed to my home phone number and picked up the phone so that she would know that I wanted her to call home for me. I didn't say anything until Eric answered the phone. Then I said, "I can say, 'Come here quick now.'" Eric started laughing because he had heard that phrase from me many times before. The poor housekeeping woman must have thought I was crazy, but I was afraid that if I said anything to her I might lose the thought and sentence in my brain.

I felt as if I had a demarcation line in the middle of my body, dividing my right side from my left. I couldn't feel my right breast. I could see that it was mine, but it felt as if it belonged to someone else.

Last night, I worked again on numbering four steps in the correct order, but trying to write the numbers by myself was very difficult. Getting the sequence right was not hard, but writing the numbers in a small space taxed me. When Donna came, she wrote the numbers for me, and that was better. I needed her deeply, as she reached out to me. I worked on solving analogies like car is to bus as helicopter is to road, cup, TV, or plane, and I got them right. Donna asked me to write my name on a sheet of paper. I had trouble with the writing, but I kept trying until I got it. I am something of a bulldozer when I want to do something, and I keep trying until I get too tired to continue. Donna also told me to get a journal.

I watched Donna when she spoke, and I hung onto every word trying to figure out how to say the word as she did.

Debbie gave me a pack of cards to pick up with my right hand. I was also working on making a circle by touching my thumb to my fingertips, one at a time.

Until I get my bearings back, I am steered around by Eric, my family, and my friends. Just sitting in bed is hard enough. Most other things I leave to them. I feel like a zombie, as if I have a glazed look in my eyes even though that might not be so. I yawn when I'm not tired. The yawns come in waves, and my days are filled with long stretches of silence.

My mind and soul are intact, even though I have trouble speaking. It seems that I have to explore for miles and miles for a word when I want to say something. Talking is appallingly difficult. At first, I made only short utterances about four words long–just fragments of a sentence. Even that took deep concentration. I was glad that Jane had been so insistent about my getting the tPA. I would not like to see what words I would be making without it. The sounds that I made before I got the drug made no sense, and I got very good at gesturing to people in order to make my needs known. One of my friends decided that I should be her partner playing charades.

Michael told me to leave the computer on since the task of turning it on was too much for me. I tried to look at letters and decide what to do with them. I could read words, but the meaning of sentences disappeared while I was reading them. Typing was inconceivable, but I was trying to relearn all that. My heart is brave, and I have to keep going on.

Eric and Jane tried to make me eat, but I was so tired that I couldn't eat much.

FROM THE SPEECH PATHOLOGIST

Once Polly could understand most of what I was saying, we went to the beginnings of pre-reading skills--the development of sound and symbol awareness, also known as phonological awareness. Polly was using a Gestalt method (seeing the whole word, not the parts) for word recognition because she could not yet break down verbal or written information into the segments that would help her decode and encode spoken and written language. I was fortunate that for a number of years I had worked with youngsters in the pre-reading stage. I was aware of what a daunting task lay ahead for Polly and of the hours and hours of repetitive, rote work that would be necessary for her to regain her phonological skills.

December 18, 1998

A problem is your chance to do your best.
Duke Ellington

The night nurses helped me to get up early and bathe before the therapists made their rounds. I'm too tired after three therapies to do anything else including bathing.

I envied people who could speak without thinking. When others were spouting a barrage of words, I felt so impotent. Words eluded me most of the time, but I spoke when people prodded me. What speech I had was abbreviated. When I said a word, it seemed to be hanging by itself on a tiny thread without any cushion for it if it fell.

Brain Attack

I couldn't seem to sort out how to do some simple tasks. When I tried to put on my socks, I had to think what I needed to do to get them on my foot. Nothing was easy, but I am one tough and driven lady. My persistence is legendary among my friends and family.

When too much information was coming at me too quickly, I got confused and my patience was nil. It helped when people repeated what I needed to do.

I liked working with Donna, but often the thought flashed in my mind: "Can I trust her without looking over my shoulder all the time?" Sometimes I looked for a way to run if I needed to. The rational part of my mind knew that the thought was irrational and was a holdover from the incident in Burlington, but I felt that way regardless. Those nurses had chipped away at my sense of safety in a hospital and at my trust in hospital personnel. I knew the incident had cast a shadow over the start of my rehab effort. It was as if my therapists were outside waiting to come in, but I couldn't let them enter.

Donna reminded me about the small victories in my day, but I failed to see them clearly. I was drained both physically and emotionally most of the time, and my heart ached.

Ana

I checked on Polly and heard that she was giving the nurses heck and teaching herself to write again. At this point I knew that good old Polly was in there and that she would climb out.

December 19, 1998

***To everything there is a season,
and a time to every purpose under the heaven.***
Ecclesiastes 3:1-2

I worked on physical therapy, but one of the things that the physical therapist wanted me to do was very difficult. I was to stand on a board called a biomechanical advantage platform and try to balance on one foot, but I never figured out what to do. Not only couldn't I do it, but the actions also didn't make sense to me.

MEDICAL FACTS

Physical therapy is used to restore the patient's mobility, which includes preservation of range of motion and re-education of motor function, coordination, balance, and gait.

From the window of my hospital room, I could see the snow outside. The beauty of the snow was as transitory as words were to me. One minute I could say a word, and in the next minute the word had disappeared from my memory.

I needed to feel safe to learn to speak again, and rehab was a refuge to me. Donna praised me for trying to talk even when it was just a gesture in response to a yes- or-no question. I liked it better if she repeated a word and said it in a sing-song way. My brain was damaged, but I didn't focus on it. I tried not to focus on the damage in my brain but on being able to speak.

When Donna told me to listen to music, I didn't do it because I couldn't do two things at the same time. If I listened to music, my coping mechanisms left me, and I started crying. I wanted to focus what little coping mechanisms I had on learning to speak. So instead of listening to music, I often sat in vacant silence.

I read an article that said that gesturing while you speak will improve your brain's recall ability. But what if one can't speak much? Does gesturing work then?

I didn't like when someone talked to me as if I was a child. I wanted only one person to talk at one time, and I didn't like having the TV on. TV was too much stimulation for me.

I was never one to take drugs, but at night my brain ached so, I took a Tylenol. It wasn't a headache, just a "brain pain."

The gravity of what happened to me was hitting home. I had lost part of myself, and I was trying valiantly to get it back. Before I had the brain attack, no signs warned "Danger!" so I blithely walked on the treadmill unaware of the risks ahead.

Mark

The stroke happened shortly before my 29th birthday, and I knew how important it was for my mother to wish me a happy birthday, but she couldn't. I was sad, not because she didn't say it but because I knew it was important to her to be able to say it to me.

FROM THE PHYSICAL THERAPIST.

Polly walked to the rehab department and managed well with her IV pole. She had difficulty balancing on the biomechanical advantage platform, but she went up and down the stairs fine.

Eric

We were fortunate to have good therapists working with Polly. It didn't take long for them to realize that she was different from most of the patients they were used to. If they told her to do something five times, she would do it ten. If they gave her a week's worth of work, they would return the next day and find it done. Polly was working day and night to get better.

December 20, 1998

Opportunities are usually disguised by hard work so most people don't recognize them.
Ann Landers

I negotiated a trip to the bathroom by myself, walking as deliberately as if I were on a high wire because I didn't want to make a mistake and fall down. I had to think about each step and then adjust it. I tried to avoid doing anything that would lengthen my hospital stay.

I had to exercise an iron discipline when I worked on trying to speak. I tried to see if I could say words, and I tried repeating a word many times to get it stuck in my mind. That took a lot of concentration. When the housekeeper came into my room, I would point to a word in a magazine and keep repeating it. When I heard her say the word, I would know if I had uttered it right.

I looked at words in a magazine article and tried to say some by myself. The words that I could say were: here, men, quit, we, eight, penny, dog, head, Polly, bed, fine, hill, beam, mother, father, doctor, dinner, no way, wind, work, meat, rain, ground, big, and women. Some of these I could say once, but not again, even though I tried. I tried and tried to say my cat's name, but I couldn't, even though her name is simple–Sugar. Some of the time I couldn't remember her name either.

With her sunny disposition, Debbie turned a bad day into a better one for me She gave me a new exercise to practice. I rested my hand on the table, spreading my fingers wide and then bringing them together. I was proud that I could tie my shoelaces.

Most of the time I was befuddled and sat staring blankly into space.

My neurologist told me that I would be able to go home as soon as my Coumadin dosage was regulated. I had been in the hospital 11 days. I was determined not to spend Christmas there. I wanted to go to my new home.

December 21, 1998

Listen to the Sounds of Silence

I wobble sometimes when I walk, but tomorrow I am going home. My physical therapists made a big deal about the stairs in my home. I didn't understand them. Didn't they know that I got down the stairs myself right after the stroke? I knew that I had many problems, but to me the stairs weren't one of them. If the worst things came to pass, I could crawl up or down.

Words are elusive creatures. I used to have a love affair with language, but instead I had a tumultuous and sometimes bitter union with words. In my mind, words were away on a sad expedition. I felt that my soul was choking. I tried to be patient, but patience is not my best suit. I wondered if the "old Polly" was still inside me.

FROM THE PHYSICAL THERAPIST

Polly was very unsteady when I woke her from a nap. She worked on walking up and down stairs, and I recommended that her husband be with her when she used the stairs at home. She will continue PT in the outpatient department after her discharge from the hospital.

Chapter Three
On With My Life

December 22, 1998

It makes all the difference whether one sees darkness through the light or brightness through the shadows.

Helen Keller

I walked out of the hospital with little help. My stubborn independence served me well.

FROM THE NEUROLOGIST--MEDICAL NOTES

Ms. Perez had a left middle cerebral artery stroke with upper extremity weakness and fine motor problems and expressive aphasia. She was treated with tPA and was transferred to the medical center where she was hospitalized for four days and transferred back to her local hospital for continued rehabilitation and neurological care.

FROM THE OCCUPATIONAL THERAPIST

Polly progressed quickly in the hospital. I was constantly having to come up with new challenges for her. She will continue her occupational therapy as an outpatient in our rehabilitation department.

December 24, 1998

I met Steve, my physical therapist for outpatient rehabilitation. The day started badly, as there was a problem scheduling my appointments, and I had to wait for him. Waiting was not a problem for me, but I wanted to be sure that I would get my full time with the therapist even though we started late. I tried and tried to communicate this thought to him, but I couldn't say the words, and I knew he didn't understand me. At last I got out the words, "You don't understand!" This wasn't the best way to meet a new therapist.

I just quit trying to explain my thoughts and started working with him. I got the feeling that he really wanted to help me. He helped me practice walking, as my steps were effortful and uncertain. I tried everything that he asked me to do. He didn't seem bothered by my anger and frustration, and he had a wonderful sense of humor. It was clear that Steve knew a lot about physical therapy and about communicating with a patient, and he wouldn't hold it against me if I was upset. I had a lot to be upset about.

I am a perfectionist. I was eager to prove to myself that I could get well and that I had enough courage and willpower to overcome the hardships that the brain attack had caused.

FROM THE PHYSICAL THERAPIST

I found out that I would get a new PT patient today. I wondered who would want to start rehab on Christmas Eve. The person who worked with Polly in the hospital told me that I would have a great person to work with, but my first impression was of an angry woman. She had had a problem with scheduling her appointments and had gotten very frustrated trying to explain it. I had trouble making sense out of what she was trying to say, but I did know that she wanted something done. When I asked what the problem was, she kept repeating, "You don't understand." I tried to let her know that I wanted to understand and help her. I did my initial exam and worked with her on some simple exercises.

It was clear that her frustration was connected to being unable to speak, and her way of dealing with the frustration was to get angry. I thought to myself, "I've got to figure out how to get inside her head and work with her."

December 25, 1998

Christmas was pathetic, as I wasn't in a very festive mood. It didn't feel like Christmas, just another day. I knew that I had to keep my strength up, but I didn't feel like eating the nice Christmas dinner that Eric and Jane made.

I was bewildered most of the day. Jane came over and helped me work on auditory and visual comparison. I could correctly identify simple objects such as a stove or a chair, but I couldn't pronounce their names. I tried to explain how the objects differed from one another.

I hated background noise, and I asked Eric to put on earphones to listen to the TV. The noise of the TV grated on my nerves and made me edgy.

I was unable to do any therapy during the Christmas vacation, and I missed talking to Donna because she helped me recognize when I improved. I practiced as much as I could without her.

December 27, 1998

Neither your past nor your present is your potential.

When I try to remember something, my thoughts seem to be short-circuited. I sound like a baby saying "want juice" instead of a full sentence. Donna told me that this is telegraphic speech. I suppose that telegraphic speech is better than no speech at all.

Donna tried to teach me how the mouth makes sounds. She told me that my lips made the letters p, b, v, t, and d; my mouth made the sounds sh, s, and z; and my throat made the letters k and g. Even though I heard what she said, her words made no sense to me. My homework was to name as many items as I could in each of 40 categories. I could name things only in seven categories: fruits (apple, pear), flowers (daisies, roses, mums, pansies, carnations, orchids, gardenias), desserts (pie), farm animals (cow), meats (hamburger), and occupations (salesman).

I couldn't read a magazine article that was continued on another page because I couldn't tell what the numbers were or find where the article continued. I read a part of many articles, but I never found out how they ended.

FROM THE PHYSICAL THERAPIST

I knew that rote exercises wouldn't work with Polly. I needed to focus on her feelings as well as on the exercises, as there wasn't much in her life that she could do. She needed to feel that she had control over something.

December 28, 1998

Any technique can become a static one-size-fits-all prescription that doesn't exactly fit anyone.

Aileen Crow

I found out that my occupational therapist was changed. The new one asked me to start all over again. Didn't she have notes about my therapy with Debbie? She said that Debbie worked only with inpatients. I asked why, and the answer was "hospital policy." I think that they should do what is best for the client and not simply follow policy. I felt that I was running in circles with the therapist change. She wanted me to be a "good patient" and submit to treatment unquestioningly, but I wanted to know everything about the rehabilitation process.

I started doing exercises with Steve. I worked on balance skills using a big physical therapy ball like the one I used with the pregnant women I taught and supported during labor in my role as a monitrice. Steve was surprised I knew about it. In my rudimentary language, I told him that I taught my pregnant clients to use the ball during pregnancy to strengthen their muscles, during labor to help the baby take the correct position for birth, and after delivery to regain stomach tone and help calm a fussy baby. Steve hadn't known about the use of the PT ball in obstetrics, and it fascinated him. And I liked being able to teach another health-care professional as I'd done for 35 years.

For my exercises Steve had me kneel on the mat, put my abdomen on the ball in front of me, and balance with my arms stretched out in front of me. Whew, was it hard for me to do!

Donna told me to find practical motor activities to do, like typing. She said that typing would strengthen my right hand and that isolated movements like needlework and writing helped too. Michael helped me with the homework Donna gave me. I tried to write words from memory by looking at a word, copying it, and then closing my eyes and writing it in the air. I didn't really get that "air writing."

December 30, 1998

*The important thing is what we are
doing not what we have to do.*
Iyengar

I was used to Debbie's making me feel good, but the new occupational therapist made me feel bad. She didn't seem to respect that I was a "whole person" not just a person to be put through her paces. She wanted me simply to follow her schedule, and this made me feel like a stick of furniture in the room.

After my day's therapies were done, I couldn't think well. My thoughts seemed hazy, as if they were covered by a veil. The saying "lost in thought" was what happened to me a lot, but I didn't even have many thoughts. I seemed to know that my thoughts were hovering in the background. I didn't realize that thinking could hurt but it did. I had "brain ache" again.

I had a "brain and mouth" problem. My brain was in the race, but my mouth wasn't. It was playing little tricks on me. The words that came out of my mouth were fractured even though the word was correct in my brain. I hoped that my mouth would catch up to my brain.

I wouldn't eat much unless Eric cooked and told me to eat, because eating wasn't important to me and I wasn't hungry. I knew I had to eat for nourishment, but I used all my energy just to speak. Sometimes, eating took too much effort.

Linda

When I found out about Polly's stroke, I sent her a light-hearted e-mail telling her that she needed some authentic Tex-Mex food, a Corona Light beer, hot Tejano music, and a Texas bluebonnet because they were better than the chicken soup that she would get up North.

FROM THE PHYSICAL THERAPIST.

I realized that Polly was tired, and I adjusted her exercise to accommodate her energy. I don't do PT as a routine that must be repeated every day. I do what the individual patient needs. Knowing that Polly was a nurse and had had her stroke while exercising on her treadmill suggested that she understood why she needed PT. As I got to know Polly better, I could tell she was goal oriented and didn't need much external motivation.

I learned quickly that Polly's PT session had to be scheduled before speech therapy because she was so beat after speech.

December 31, 1998

If you have faith as a mustard seed , you will say to this mountain, "Move from here to there" and nothing will be impossible for you.
Matthew 17:20

I left occupational therapy in tears again. I needed a person who treated me like a thinking individual. The therapist was annoyed every time I asked her a question.

In speech therapy, I looked at a picture for one minute and tried to answer questions about what things were in it. Donna explained that the exercise was meant to show how I was looking at the picture.

No longer could I recognize what the numbers in my checkbook signified. I knew what they were meant to say, but the amount of money I had in the bank was an enigma.

Brain Attack

I had to remember that only three weeks had passed since the brain attack. I shouldn't have been discouraged with what I had accomplished. I still had in my mind the saying, "It's good enough for government work," and that was how I felt when I spoke. I was on an uphill path to speaking; instead I wanted to be bounding up the steps to jabbering again.

There was no shortcut to learning to talk again. If I tried to say something, only a few words came out. I had trouble remembering a sentence until I finished it, and I needed assistance searching for the word that I wanted to say. I waited for words in the same way storm chasers anticipate the next tornado. When other people spoke, the words came our in a blur of speed; when I said words, they came out at a glacial pace.

Tonight when I was having dinner in a restaurant, the waitress was spinning out a litany of choices and specials. I watched how easily she said words. Her words seemed to wash over me like water from a waterfall. I got so much pleasure in that.

Jane and I talked to the two doctors on my case this week. We wanted to know why the ER doctor hadn't told my family and me about tPA until Jane mentioned it several times. They said that the doctor had mentioned it, but Jane insisted that the doctor didn't even broach the subject. They remained evasive, so I asked again. The excuse they gave was a combination of fear of lawsuits and politics between the medical center and the rural hospital. In my halting words, I asked what would have happened if Jane had not been there. They had no answer for that. I guess I wouldn't be speaking at all. That's a scary thought, as most people who have a stroke don't have an advocate like Jane with them in the ER.

I told my son who calls me every day to talk to me "normally," and I found that I could understand him.

Most of the time I find no pleasure in eating, and I have trouble deciding what to eat.

I feel an inner force propelling me forward, and sometimes I get anxious because I don't know what would come next.

A.P. and Theda (Parents)

Paulina was working hard to improve herself. Since we called her every week, we noticed that she could communicate better in the morning after a restful night's sleep than she could in the afternoons or evenings when she was tired.

Chapter Four
The Start of the Last Year of the Century

January 1, 1999

Everyone must row with the oars she has.
English Proverb

I started the year in an almost wordless world, and I didn't like it any way I saw it. The almost-mute world felt cold and lonely. I couldn't gather my thoughts or the answers to questions fast enough. I decided that I might be able to write down some words that I could see in my mind, and I did succeed in writing them, but all of this baffled me. I didn't know why.

Donna told me I might be helped by writing down the names of people I knew because I could make an association from the person to the written word, so I copied the 407 names in my address book.

I worked on saying the appropriate word that would complete a sentence and then on naming objects such as table, couch, tree, and toilet. I couldn't spell most of the words, even though they weren't very hard.

I know that my life will not be like it was before, but what will it be like?

Sue

I seriously considered giving up public speaking about obstetrics when I heard about Polly's stroke. Knowing the impact Polly's lectures have had on changing obstetrical practices across the country, I felt that I had lost a valuable friend and colleague. Hearing from Polly's husband that she was working hard to learn to speak again was humbling and made me reflect about what we consider valuable. What I realized was that we all have been given gifts, but it is up to us to use them. I felt that if I was able to make a difference in the health care of women, I had to respect that gift as long as I had it. Polly's stroke taught me that.

Brain Attack

January 2, 1999

Decide what you want;
decide what you are willing to exchange for it.
Establish your priorities and go to work.

H. L. Hunt

Two friends phoned me. I could understand them, and to my surprise they had no trouble understanding me either. Perhaps I am getting better.

I admit that the stress I was under for the six months before the brain attack must have contributed to the stroke because there was nothing wrong with my heart and other blood vessels. Obviously my blood has the tendency to clot easily. Did I do this to myself? Did I create my own wordless hell?

Michael was helping with my computer work by telling me the words to type from a list the speech therapist had given me. That was part of my homework for Donna.

In the evening I read a descriptive paragraph and then decided whether statements about it were true or false. That was easy. Then I worked on visual scanning – looking at a group of numbers and crossing out the numbers that didn't belong. To practice sequencing, I had to put in order the steps to many things, but most of the time my brain seemed as fuzzy as a peach.

When people estimate how long it will take me to resume my profession, I think to myself that I can recover faster. They just didn't know me. In my brain the words "I can do anything" reverberate all the time. I will repeat that phrase until I can be a public speaker again.

FROM THE SPEECH PATHOLOGIST

I encouraged Polly to copy words on paper, type them on a computer, and say the words aloud. She experienced profound frustration with saying parts of two words at the same time (as she was later able to describe it) with the constant result that the "middles" of words seemed to be missing.

January 3, 1999

The great thing in this world is not so much where we are but in what direction we are moving.
Oliver Wendell Holmes

My speech is a motley crew of mangled words. My voice sounds peculiar to me, and what speech I have is tremendously effortful, the opposite of the quick way I used to speak. I have to think hard to say anything at all. I have no time to worry about how I sound as saying a word is hard enough. Most of the people I talk to know that I had a stroke, but strangers probably think that I'm "slow." That doesn't bother me. It's their problem.

I feel forlorn and in an odd way lucky too. I'm lucky to be alive even if I'm "damaged." Sometimes when I can't talk right, even though I'm trying the best that I can, I feel discouraged. Frustration is a demon I could live without. My spirit feels imprisoned.

It's hard to tell if I'm getting better when I don't have sessions with the rehab team for a few days. Time passes more slowly when I can't assess my progress every day. I have glimpses of how I used to speak, but most of the time I try not to think about it.

I worked on the computer, writing down words from memory and then typing them on the computer. I had trouble remembering where letters were on the keyboard. I wrote a rudimentary e-mail message to my mom and dad, although I had trouble spelling and typing. Then I printed the message out. It contained two sentences: "Thank your for calling. I like you to calling me."

I continued to do needlepoint to try to make my right hand work better.

January 4, 1999

Listen to what the experts say, but always rely on your own judgement.
Albert Einstein

Over the weekend, I made the wrenching decision to stop working with my current occupational therapist. I told Donna that I knew my decision would lengthen my rehab. She asked me if I wanted to keep working in OT, and I told her I did but only if there was a change of therapists. I felt better once I had made the decision. I always felt humiliated after the OT sessions. When I couldn't understand something, the therapist seemed to be scolding me. Debbie was so cheerful and positive, but the new therapist often made me feel that I was doing something wrong. She never treated me like a partner in my own rehabilitation. If the other therapists did something that didn't work, they tried something different. I wanted a therapist who would treat me like a whole person and see me and not just my disabilities.

I knew our working relationship needed to be a team effort, but I didn't have the strength to be the one to build the team. The therapist had no desire to make our relationship work except on her terms. I am a teacher at heart, and although I wanted to explain to her how to work with me, I never did. If I were well, I could probably have helped her understand, but I couldn't do it. I struggled with this episode in my rehab journey. I was used to being the caregiver; receiving care was hard for me.

I gave Donna the 16 homework sheets that I had done. I felt that I didn't have anything to lose by doing them. I had toiled on crossword puzzles and exercises to make my handwriting better. The handwriting looked like mine again. I had been practicing writing names in my day timer. I had been forced into a new relationship with my brain. Donna told me that I was working on improving my motor-planning skills–getting out the words that were in my mind.

I was really tired during the day and it was hard to do physical therapy. I worked with Steve on a scissor-like gait where I repeatedly crossed one leg over another. It confused me sometimes.

January 5, 1999

Michael helped me type words from the cards that Donna lent me. I copied and typed 237 words in one day. I also typed words for each letter of the alphabet even though I kept forgetting what letter of the alphabet came next. It feels that I can't do much right.

Affirmations are just spoken imagery, and I kept telling myself that I would speak again. I felt that I didn't have anything to lose by doing that.

I had to build a bridge over the gap between my mind and my mouth. In my brain the words were correct, but when I tried to speak, jumbled-up sounds emerged from my mouth. Where do the words get detoured?

Every time I start to talk, I think my speech will be fine, but that rarely happens. Language bubbles inside of me but can't get out of my mouth. I would spend every bit of my money if I could make words flow easily from my mouth.

I refuse to be a victim. I am a survivor.

FROM THE PHYSICAL THERAPIST.

Polly seemed less tired, so we worked on balance exercises. Her strength is increasing, and with each new exercise she asks, "Why are you having me do this?" I know that Polly needs more detailed information than most of my stroke clients.

January 6, 1999

Donna coaxed and cajoled me to try to say words. My homework was to name a word for the first 17 letters of the alphabet, and I came up with these words: apple, boat, cat, dog, each, folk, go, hand, idea, Jello, know, lasso, memo, neon, open, and peony. I had trouble with the words boat and peony, as I couldn't understand what letter was between "O" and "T" in boat and the letter between ""O" and "Y" in peony. I often can't spell the middle of the word. I have to ask Eric all the time what letter completes the word.

When Steve told me to do something 12 times, I would do 13. I told him that the other one was for good measure.

January 7, 1999

Show me the path where I should go,
point the right road for me to walk.
Lead me; teach me.
Psalm 25:4-5

The head therapist was consulted about my refusal to work in OT with my present therapist, and she decided to send me back to Debbie, the first OT therapist that I had in the hospital..The head therapist must have understood what was important to my healing. I was thankful that she knew that I needed to play a central role in my own treatment.

With a team of people concerned about my welfare, I feel that I am coming home. Now that we are working together and respect each other, I know I have a good chance of getting better and helping my poor, sick brain.

Debbie taught me an exercise called wall push-ups. I placed my hands at shoulder height and shoulder-width apart on a wall and stepped back until my arms were fully extended. Then I slowly bent my elbows until my chest was a few inches from the wall. Keeping my back straight and my abdominal muscles tight and squeezing my chest muscles, I pushed away from the wall to straighten my arms. I had to do about 12 repetitions.

I worked on bridging exercises to strengthen my back and legs. I lay on my back with my feet flat on the floor, hip-width apart about a foot from my buttocks. I pressed my feet into the floor and lifted my pelvis until my body was a straight line from my knees to my shoulders. Pregnant women are often given a similar exercise to strengthen their back and stomach muscles. Steve told me that bridging also helped eliminate hyperextension of my knees by strengthening my quadriceps, the muscles in the front of the thighs. I tried to hold the bridge position for 30 seconds, but that was hard to do.

I worked on ordering information again, and I was learning to use compensatory strategies like a mental crutch. One strategy was to look at the first letter of a word in my mind or on a page and think about how the letter sounded. I hope that I'll progress from crutches to braces and eventually to talking on my own. I'm sure not ready to run a word marathon yet.

I wish that the brain attack hadn't happened, but what good would complaining about it do?

FROM THE PHYSICAL THERAPIST

Polly can't feel much on the outside of her right leg.

January 8, 1999

Have you had a good laugh lately?

Rehab forms a cocoon that insulates me from the outside world. I worked with Steve doing more bridging with the ball to strengthen my back and legs. To make the exercise harder, I had to do it with one leg extended in front of me. I also did wall slides where I put the ball between my back and the wall, bent my knees, and slowly slid down the wall.

Debbie and I worked on addition. Donna and Debbie thought that I knew the answers to the problems, but I wasn't sure; I guess I just had to trust them. You might think that you couldn't find anything funny in rehab, but we laughed lot. Some days, I cracked up when I wanted to say something and the word came out wrong. Donna was looking for the things that might help me use the accessible parts of my brain. Sometimes the only way to get over a hurdle is to have a good sense of humor.

Part of my homework was to read a directive and write the word it asked for. The exercise was so hard, I could do only three out of 20. The three I could do were:

Think of something bigger than a goldfish. I wrote "dog."

Think of something higher than a flagpole. I wrote "buid," *but I meant building.*

Think of something older than a toddler. I wrote "man."

I had to come to grips with my new life. I couldn't trust my instincts anymore.

I devoted many hours to speaking again, until my body said "enough" and I went to sleep.

FROM THE PHYSICAL THERAPIST

Polly commented that she sees that I like my job. I had fun working with her today. Our working relationship is solid, even though it got off to a rocky start. She pedaled on the Nu-step exercise machine for 15 minutes at level 4 and worked on single leg bridging with and without the ball.

Dee

When Polly, my favorite nursing student, wrote to me about her stroke, her handwriting was uneven and she left letters and words unfinished. Some thoughts ended in mid-sentence, but she did make sense.

The content was typically "Polly." I could feel her frustration and her determination to overcome this dastardly disability. She seemed to be challenging her body, "How dare you do this to me!"

59

Chapter Five
Sink or Swim

Month Two

January 9, 1999

By the end of the first month, I knew that I was in the best of hands with my rehab team of Debbie, Donna, and Steve. I still felt like a boat bobbing on an ocean, but I trusted that these three people would not let me sink.

I worked on answering questions about number groups. I had to look at a group of numbers and decide which one didn't belong. Doing that drained my energy.

With being unable to talk, my identity narrowed to a small groove.

My attempts at speaking resembled a bull playing in a china shop, and my apraxia kept knocking down things. My words were tangled in a weedy undergrowth in my mind. I was grateful that I had someone to help me uncover them. I learned from Donna that I was working on cortical reorganization: I would change how my brain functioned or die trying.

There were spaces in my thoughts where a truck could drive through.

<u>Mark</u>

I called my mom every day for awhile because I knew how important it was to keep her spirits up and to let her know that she was getting better every day.

At first, the fact that she couldn't communicate verbally was shocking. It is still strange to hear from an earlier voice-mail message how she sounded before the stroke. I wasn't scared that she wouldn't talk again. I almost took for granted that she would make herself better, and I was surprised that some people didn't think she would.

January 10, 1999

There's only one corner of the universe you can be certain of improving and that's your own self.

Aldous Huxley

I was working on counting by tens, but saying the words was very difficult. I tried to name objects, but I missed some, and I couldn't spell the words right. I could spell the beginning of the word and the ending of the word but the middle was still lost.

I wrote on powder a lot to learn to spell. Both my occupational therapist and my speech therapist told me that powder writing helped because there was a connection from my brain to my finger. It was the first thing that I could do by myself. I also typed about 30 words and named some words for each letter of the alphabet.

Debbie told me to rub the right side of my body with brushes of varying textures, and she gave me four weight-bearing exercises to increase sensation and body awareness. I was supposed to lean my body against a wall, lie down on my right side on a bed or couch, lean on my right elbow and forearm on a bed or couch, and also get down on all fours.

Sometimes I still have the feeling that there has been a terrible mistake, for what did I do to deserve this? I think that I look sad most of time, or so it feels to me. This experience is lonely. In some respects, it's like giving birth. When I gave birth to my children, others were around me to help me, but the job was mine, and in some ways it was lonely too.

FROM THE OCCUPATIONAL THERAPIST

Polly was willing to try anything. For example, I spread baby powder on a table so she could write with her right index finger the words that she couldn't say. Her fine motor control was not re-developed enough to write easily with a pen. When I replaced the pen with powder, she could write!

January 11, 1999

You must do the thing you think you cannot do.
Eleanor Roosevelt

The day was not enjoyable because I had a tough time getting anything to work right. Everything was confusing. Trying to speak was my idea of hell. Words seemed to be burned up before I could say them. Saying any word was grueling and drawn out. I tried to locate words in a puzzle. I got 23 words right and couldn't find 16. Well, I got more right than wrong. I didn't want to wallow in self-pity, but I had trouble telling myself to "suck it up," and that never used to a problem for me.

I started to work on addition, but I could do little. Numbers didn't make sense to me. I could add single digit numbers, but for answers greater than 10, I needed help. 7 plus 8 was beyond me.

January 12, 1999

A word after a word after a word is power.
Margaret Atwood

The source of my agony is not apparent until I speak. When people in the "outside world" hear me, my speech deficits frighten them.

I still have trouble saying words, so I'm not sure I'm getting better. It's amazing what my mind goes through just to say a simple word. My sentences are rudimentary, I omit articles and prepositions, and use only the present tense. I am impatient when I can't say what I want to.

The aphasia piqued my intellectual curiosity, and I wanted to know why I couldn't talk. Many of my speech sessions began with the word "why." I needed to know more about my brain so that I could understand the wanderings of the words I wanted to say.

My homework was to talk about my favorite parts of my profession. I wrote that I like helping women find strength they didn't know they had. The other part I like is enabling babies to be born without obstetrical drugs in their systems.

It was easy to get confused, and I couldn't do an exercise that Debbie asked me to do. You might think that slapping both hands on your knees, clapping your hands together, and then snapping your fingers would be easy but I kept forgetting what to do next. I knew what I needed to do but remembering the right order was another matter.

Brain Attack

Often I sit gazing out of the window of my house. The view never ceases to captivate me. Where I live is a dream of rural peace. The scene that I see through my living room window must have evolved over the years, and the thought of that amazes me. The way the countryside was forever changing seemed to parallel my life.

FROM THE PHYSICAL THERAPIST

Polly worked on agility drills and cross-over shuttle steps. Her gait was smoother, but she had trouble distinguishing her right side from her left. With most people, I have to ask if the skill is getting easier, but not with Polly. She would tell me about an exercise, "This is easy now."

January 13, 1999

Growth demands a temporary surrender of security.
Gail Sheehy

I talked to a good friend from Houston who is a midwife, and that brightened my day. I told her that some days I felt that I would like to have an epidural (the regional anesthetic often given to women in labor in a hospital) for this rehab process. She told me that I was having a homebirth for my rehab (meaning no anesthetics), and she would be my midwife.

When I wrote, I tried to hold on to the essence of the sentence in my mind, but my mind was constantly fragmented, and I lost the sentence somewhere most of the time. After I wrote a sentence, I filled in the small words (such as in, one, and of) later, and this worked better for me than trying to write the sentence perfectly from the start.

The progress in my therapy is measured in baby steps, not leaps and bounds. I kept in my head some correspondence that I wanted to write, but the letters seemed to be stuffed in an old drawer. I wanted to be able to send the correspondence via real words, not just through thoughts in my mind.

I still can't feel most of my right side, and it seems that it doesn't exist even though I can see it.

January 14, 1999

Resolve to be thyself: and know,
that he who finds himself, loses his misery.
Mathew Arnold

I reached a milestone: I started writing in my journal by myself instead of dictating it to Eric.

I want my old self to reemerge. I can't remember anymore what normal is. I worked on exercises for my memory, and I eagerly awaited signs of improvement. The things that used to take little or no effort now take concerted effort.

Not a day goes by that I don't ask myself, "Why did those nurses in ward six in Burlington treat me so badly?" The episode repeats in my mind like a kaleidoscope turning and turning. I hope those haunting and taunting memories will go away,

Some days I think that my speech sounds more like myself, and then I feel that I am getting better. I was beginning to type my e-mails myself, and I wanted to use my treadmill again. The get-well cards that I received, especially from people I didn't know, helped greatly. I'm amazed that people took time out of their day to send me notes, cards, and packages.

I have never been so tired, and I feel like a limp dishrag a lot of the time. Because of the exhaustion, I cry easily. More than once my tears have turned into semi-hysterical sobbing, and I am inconsolable until exhaustion overcomes me.

January 15, 1999

Life is a grindstone.
But whether it grinds us down or polishes us up depends on us.

L. Thomas Holdcroft

I asked Steve if I could start using my treadmill again so he checked me out on it and told me that I could start using it at home once again.

After looking at these phrases only once, I typed them from memory on the computer one at a time.

Blink your eyes.	Write a letter.	Help me up.
Write a letter.	Eat the lunch.	Hang up the phone.
When are we leaving?	Walk the dog.	How is your friend?
What does that mean?	How are you?	What time is it?
Answer the phone.	Where is the car?	Who is that man?
When did you go?	Open the door.	Wash your hands.
Give me your hand.	Sign your name.	Read a book.
Walk the dog.	How are you?	What is your name?

After I typed the exercise I was so tired; I have little residual strength to draw on.

A doctor friend from Houston sent me information about hormone therapy after a stroke, which was more detailed than what I had already received. We had worked together, and he knew that I needed and could understand more information than the average patient. I don't do well with pat answers. The doctor I'm seeing here doesn't understand that about me yet.

Steve's charm and humor was what I needed today. He made me laugh even though I didn't have anything to laugh about.

FROM THE PHYSICAL THERAPIST

Polly asked when she could start using her treadmill again. She walked on the treadmill at 1.8 mph for five minutes and will start doing it at home too. When I work with Polly, I always explain the "why" of therapy because she wants to be able to decide what she will do, although she has never refused to try anything I asked.

January 16, 1999

Flagging spirits.

I didn't feel very good because my head felt funny, and I couldn't think or talk as well as I could yesterday. I wish that I could speak fluently like I used to. I just want my life back, please.

Even though I didn't feel good, I made a brochure on the computer for one of our products.

I went to bed to escape into sleep so I wouldn't break into a rage of tears and frustration again.

MEDICAL FACTS

Post-stroke emotions are part of adjusting to the changes brought on by the stroke. Some psychological reactions to stroke are: frustration, anxiety, anger, apathy, depression, and lack of motivation.

January 18, 1999

Craving control over my words.

I don't think that I will ever be able to speak as I used to. I have to make tremendous personal and social adjustments. Individuals often act around me as if I don't know what's happening. While I still have trouble thinking logically sometimes, I am fully aware of my problems.

I practiced typing the following phrases:

Open the door	Wash your hands	Read a book
Walk the dog	Help me up	Give me your hand
Sign your name	Answer the phone	It's time to go

I could type some of the phrases the first time that I tried, but others took more attempts. My brain spun with the phrases that I typed. This exercise was very hard.

Once in a while, I get a click of awareness of how my life used to be, and that saddens me.

Brain Attack

January 20, 1999

The greater the obstacle, the more glory in overcoming it.
Jean-Baptiste Moliéré

My homework was to look at some sentences for a few seconds and then type them without looking at the text. The exercise was designed to improve my memory. It took a long time to type a simple list.

I have private conversations with myself in my head. Without words, I have no way to unburden my heart to others.

Celeste

My husband had a stroke nine years ago, and I contacted Polly to offer my help. I am a nurse too--Polly and I have been colleagues for many years--and the best advice I could give her was not to believe most of what the doctors and nurses said about limits on her recovery. My husband still continues to improve.

January 23, 1999

You have to expect things of yourself before you can do them.
Michael Jordan

I practiced typing 84 words today and worked on unscrambling words and syllables. My homework also included completing familiar phrases, such as "As blind as a ____." Eric had to help me with that one.

I used visualization to help me say words. I tried to see in the theater of my mind the words that I wanted to say.

Eric

I have always been someone who rolls with the punches. I knew that as long as I could see in Polly's eyes that she was functioning mentally, she would be okay eventually. We were in this together. It was as if we were in school together, but I was further along than Polly so I had to help her catch up.

January 25, 1999

Language is the light of the mind.
John Suart Mill

I labored on combining simple sentences to make compound sentences and on outlining steps for common activities. That stuff was hard.

Sometimes the word I wanted to say got stuck in my mouth like a phonograph needle in a cracked record, and I just kept repeating the same thing. Apraxia was like going the wrong way down a one-way street.

My exhaustion had a raw edge to it like a torn fabric. Tiredness made me so ragged, I felt that I could cry at the least provocation.

<u>FROM THE SPEECH PATHOLOGIST</u>

Within six weeks, Polly was speaking, reading, writing, and spelling simple words and phrases. She was improving daily with lightning speed. I would tell her to do one page of work, knowing full well that she would do five or more. As we worked so closely together that first month, I realized that I had met a very special woman. We worked well together in a professional relationship, but we also shared much in our lives and interests. I felt a tremendous burden of responsibility for this woman, as if I had to be sure that she would recover sufficiently to be able to go back to her profession. That was potentially not a healthy position for me as a therapist, and I knew that. I had to remind myself repeatedly that I was a therapist and facilitator and that I didn't possess "magic fairy dust" (as I said to Polly's father) to make her all better. That would have made life so simple. I have never met such a determined individual.

January 28, 1999

I worked on identifying times and events using common items, such as *"A shotput is used at _____ [track meets]."* I also practiced identifying things by class, origin, function, location, composition, critical elements, or attributes. The amount of energy that I had to spend on a task like that was amazing.

Brain Attack

FROM THE PHYSICAL THERAPIST

Polly occasionally lost her balance and fell backward when she worked with the green ball, but she was aware of it. It's important to her safety that she knows when something is wrong.

January 29, 1999

Great works are performed, not by strength, but perseverance.

Samuel Johnson

My homework was to define words by their composition. I had to complete sentences telling what each thing was made of, such as *"A roof is made of _____ [tin]."* I did all but one of 50 sentences. The one that eluded me was *"Pie crusts are made of ____."* I couldn't think of anything to finish the sentence.

January 31, 1999

Words mean more than what is set down on paper.
It takes the human voice to infuse
them with shades of deeper meaning.

Maya Angelou

I can't hear the difference between the word "pay" and the word "say." To relearn, I worked diligently to say these words over and over again: bay, bee, by, bow, boo. Saying those five words took me a long time.

I tried to list as many everyday things as I could, such as bathroom and paper products and cutting utensils, but I could think of only three items. I worked on saying the word "barbecue" and completed sentences by filling in blanks with appropriate adjectives. I also wrote about where I live.

I wrote...

"I live in a house that faces a tall mountain. It has four levels and four bedrooms plus a tiny room for my treadmill. We have our offices for Cutting Edge Press and Childbirth and Family Education there. One we were working when a moose walked right read the house. Deer saunter in our back yard a lot.

This is a lot different from where we used to live. There were approximately 50,000 in the subdivision. It was hot there most of the time. It never was wither there but it was summer of if te time. Our air conditioning bill was high even when we used all of our ceiling fans."

I wrote a Valentine letter to all the people who sent cards to me. Composing the letter took a long time, but I kept thinking about the adage, "If at first you don't succeed, try, try again." I love hearts, and Valentine's Day is my favorite holiday after Christmas. In the letter, I thanked my friends for the cards, presents, and flowers they sent me and which brightened many of my days. I told my friends that I worked hard every day so that I could spell, add, subtract, and divide.

I wanted to escape from the effort of thinking and the hard work of concentration. Before the stroke, I never thought about what my brain was doing while I was concentrating. Now I realize how much is involved in thinking.

Donna went to a seminar on animal communication yesterday. I told her that I was just working on human communication, but if communication with animals was easier, maybe I should change.

Donna has a sharp mind, and in some ways she reminds me of myself. I wonder if I will ever have a sharp mind again.

Chapter Six
My War With Words

February 1, 1999

I will survive.

The Grateful Dead

I worked on finding words that I would need to use in conversational speech. I had trouble retrieving the word that I wanted to use.

Donna told me that my struggle with words was a little like dyslexia even though I can read all right. I can read complex material, but I can't say the words I'm reading. I stumble over new words, as if the wiring in my brain was scrambled. Donna will help me rewire the part of my brain that forms words. I have so much to relearn, beginning with distinguishing real spoken words from the nonsense that often comes out of my mouth.

Donna's homework for my brain was to type some free associations. This was hard but fun because the categories were fuzzy things, slimy things, happy things, scary things, and annoying things.

Sometimes I am fascinated by the workings of my brain, but other times I feel like a fly caught forever in a spider web. Words get scrambled on the way from my brain to my lips. I want to receive a postcard from the words in my head telling me how they're doing. My mouth is lonely without them. Words were my constant companion for more than 50 years, and I miss them. I hope they're on vacation, not gone for good.

I figure that my job right now is rehab. I have three therapy sessions at the hospital every day and then I work at home every evening. That takes so much out of me. At night the fog in my brain is so thick that I can't concentrate enough to even watch TV.

The messages from my on-line friends have helped me stay afloat in a sea of emotions. A message I received today told me that my friends were with me, if not in person, then in spirit.

FROM THE PHYSICAL THERAPIST.

Polly's gait was better today, and she worked on agility drills, bridging, and single-limb balancing. Polly's personality is to keep working no matter what. I often see that she wants to say something but can't, and this frustrates her no end.

FROM THE OCCUPATIONAL THERAPIST.

With her eyes covered, Polly could use her right hand to discriminate and correctly name five textures. The loss of protective sensation has returned and is now normal. She was 100 percent accurate in identifying ten objects including coins with her right hand while she was blindfolded. She often "bumps into doorways" with the right side of her body as her proprioception, or body awareness, was only 50 percent accurate. Her ability to tell time was improved, but she wasn't able to make change for money accurately. In tests of her cognition, she was 100 percent accurate for simple, written problems, but she was unable to complete two-step word problems. She can write words with 80 percent accuracy, but 20 percent of the words had gaps in the middle. She still had difficulty with the letter r. She uses writing to compensate for her speech deficits. Polly started using the computer, but she reported having difficulty finding the right keys on the keyboard.

February 2, 1999

I received an e-mail from an obstetrician friend telling me that he was sorry that the brain work was so hard. He said that the labor that I was doing was helping my progress, and he was sorry he couldn't give me oxytocin [a drug that brings on labor contractions] for my work.

I began thinking about the possibility of writing an article that would depict the views of a stroke client and a speech therapist, even though my words were lying below the frozen soil, covered by winter snow.

A doula (a woman who assists women during labor and after delivery) in Connecticut sent me a guided imagery to use with my work in rehab. I used guided imagery in childbirth classes to teach mothers-to-be to relax and focus. While music plays, someone quietly reads about a place like the one in the image my friend sent. The women lie down with their eyes closed, clear their minds, let go of tension, and picture themselves in the imagined place.

"You are standing on a silent road at the edge of an empty beach. There are no people in sight, and you are alone. With your eyes closed, you raise your head toward the sun, high in the blue sky, and feel its warmth on your face. The sun's rays erase all your worries, your tension, your distraction. There is only you and the beach before you....

You slowly move forward to the edge on the sand. You remove your shoes and are now barefoot. As you step into the sand, feel it on your feet. It is soft and loose, and warm and dry. It feels comforting to your skin and you sink as you step.

You stand still for a moment, to experience your surroundings. The day is fair and bright. There is a light, warm breeze that moves in little swirls around your body. It moves through your hair and your clothes and allows you to feel free and unrestrained.

You can smell the seashore and you hear seagulls a short distance away. Feel the sun's rays on your head and your back, between your shoulders.

Listen to the gentle waves as they move along the edge of the sand. Watch them roll in and out, in rhythm with your breathing. You move closer to the water's edge. Feel the sand under your feet as it becomes firmer and cooler. Now your feet don't sink into the sand but leave little moist puddles as you step. The cool wetness seeps between your toes.

You move to the edge of the water, and it washes your feet. The water is a perfect temperature for your body. You step slowly deeper, and you are aware of the waves caressing your body.

You lean forward into the water and realize that you can float and let the rhythm of the ocean rock you. You are totally relaxed and moving with the water's motion. You are supported effortlessly. You are at peace."

I was always good at visualization, so I used my friend's imagery to help me feel peaceful. I don't feel peace much anymore.

February 4, 1999

FROM THE PHYSICAL THERAPIST.

It was very busy in the clinic, and I couldn't give Polly as much time as I wanted. She is motivated enough not to let this bother her, and she worked independently. Some clients you have to be on all the time, but with Polly it wasn't a problem. I observed Polly squatting to pick up an item from the floor. Since squatting changes the body's center of gravity, being able to squat meant that her balance skills have improved.

February 8, 1999

Testing our relationship

I had no homework for the weekend, so I started to read a book for the first time since the brain attack. Writing is getting easier, so I sent short e-mails. I had problems trying to decide what to write and retrieving the words I needed. I looked at the pages that I did in the hospital and realized that I was improving. It will be a long time before I can write books again, though.

The week got off to a lousy start. I didn't feel like talking, and I didn't know why. I had to go to speech therapy, and when Donna asked how I felt, I answered, "Okay." When she asked me another question, the reply was the same, "Okay." This continued through several more questions, and my answer was always, "Okay." Then Donna asked me, "Would you bullshit me?" I said, "Probably." With that, I knew that Donna was dependable, and at last I had a feeling of utter trust in her. Our exchange helped to break down the wall that I had erected because of the way I had been treated at the medical center hospital. Until then, there had been only a fragile trust between us. From then on, we both knew that we could confront each other and trust each other. It was a breakthrough for both of us.

February 9, 1999

Don't be satisfied with stories about how things have gone with others. Unfold your own myth.

Rumi

Steve is a model of optimism. I need that so much, as I know what I want to say, but the right words don't come out. The words I want to say are broken like a mirror even though the reflections of the words in my mind are still as beautiful as they used to be

I spent a lot of time hunched over my homework like a school child. My homework tonight was working with number groups and fractions, percentages, and decimals. Numbers are a confusing entity to me now. I used to be very good at math, and I can't even subtract now. I also worked on answering common questions with numbers, understanding addition and subtraction words, and using a calendar. My all-consuming need was to learn any math concept, but it was exhausting and futile.

I felt sad for Eric, as I was often crabby. Talking takes so much effort that I have no patience left.

Eric

I knew how hard Polly was working, so I understood why she was often cantankerous. I would have been worse.

Robin

Polly and I communicated in person, via the phone, and over the Internet. After her stroke we were able to communicate only by phone at first. She was trying to remember the word for what she did. I listened as she tried, "Nurk, nurk, you know what I went to school for!" She was very persistent, and at last she said the word "nurse."

FROM THE PHYSICAL THERAPIST

Polly verbalized her frustration with trying to talk by saying, "I know what I want to say, but it's tormenting me that I can't say the words I want." I tried to figure out what she wanted to say but sometimes it was difficult as she had only rudimentary speech, her thought patterns weren't clear, and she couldn't give me many clues. I wanted her to know that I would be patient enough for her to express her thoughts.

February 11, 1999

It's helped to set dreams and never ever give up.
Florence Griffith Joyner

In my speech therapy sessions, I discussed situations that might produce the following feelings in a person: excited, angry, bored, annoyed, happy, tired, disappointed, relaxed, nasty, hopeful, worried, sympathetic, terrified, cautious, grateful, isolated, surprised, nervous, and sad. This was not easy to do. I had to search for a word that would describe the situation, but often I couldn't come up with a word and I also had trouble forming the sounds I needed to say the word. The exercise left me feeling frustrated.

A friend wrote me that her husband was an occupational therapist and had been describing a typical stroke recovery process to her so she would know what I am going through. The note helped me know that others understand how difficult this is. I am not alone.

Brain Attack

Pamela

When I called Polly, her attitude was amazingly positive. Many stroke patients I have worked with were depressed. But then Polly is a fighter and a plucky one, too.

February 13, 1999

We learn the rope of life by untying its knots.
Jean Toomer

Today my homework consisted of eight pages. In one, I answered the question "What qualities are important in a friend?" The qualities I wrote down were love, kindness, sweetness, empathy, loyalty, sympathy, and will defend me if needed. Next I worked on a deduction puzzle using clues to figure out what language people in the puzzle spoke, what sport they played, and what they did for a living. It was hard, but I kept at it until I figured it out. I also worked on word deduction to determine what object was being described by three clue words. That one wasn't very hard. I read a paragraph and answered questions about it. I breezed through that one in record time. Next, I defined a word and made a sentence using it, such as "Gymnasts have to be limber to do flips." I also completed 20 thoughts by filling in the words that completed the thought. An analogy exercise required a lot of thought to complete, but I finally did it too.

I felt drab. My reserves were depleted quickly, and I was so tired by the end of the day.

There is no fun in my life. I feel isolated, separate, and alone most of the time.

Cheri

When I talked to Polly, she sounded much better than I had anticipated. Her speech was slow, and she sometimes had to ask her husband for the word she wanted to say. One word she was trying to retrieve was "hospital." It was daunting to hear her speak about relearning to count and working in a first-grade workbook. Talking to Polly let me know she was okay, but she had a long way to go in her rehab effort.

February 14, 1999

Plunge boldly into the thick of life.
Johann Wolfgang van Goethe

The functional memory task and paragraph retention exercises went easily, and I could compare objects by stating how they were similar in size, composition, function, color, texture, smell, sound, and shape, as in "How are a car and a truck alike?" I did some of my homework on the computer. Typing took longer than writing in long hand, but I kept at it.

A friend of mine sent me an article telling about therapy with amphetamines for stroke patients. I checked it out, but I don't like to take drugs, so that therapy didn't appeal to me. It was a good article, because it showed the neurophysiology of strokes – what happens to the nerves that makes strokes so destructive.

MEDICAL FACTS

There are many new studies and therapies for stroke on the horizon. Dr. Hal Unwin and colleagues reported on the use of amphetamines to accelerate the rate of recovery for certain stroke patients.

UT SouthwesternSwmed.edu

Dr. James Grotta of the University of Texas in Houston found that a relatively small amount of coffee and the equivalent of about one drink of alcohol a day given up to two hours after a stroke reduced damage to the brain by 80 percent in animals.

Intelhealth.com

Drs. Maria Perez Barreto and Annlia Paganini-Hill of the University of Southern California in Los Angeles reported that current users of estrogen replacement therapy (HRT) had a 30 percent lower risk of developing stroke-inducing blood clots to the brain than non-users.

Intelhealth.com

Doctors at the University of Texas in Houston and at the Cleveland Clinic have studied the effect of dropping the stroke victim's temperature a few degrees for a day or so to stop the destruction of brain cells

From research at Cleveland Clinic and UT at Houston

Bryan

The handwriting on the letter in my mailbox looked like my mother's writing but cleaner. It was bizarre that her handwriting could get better after the stroke. The brain is a weird thing.

February 15, 1999

A problem is your chance to do your best.
Duke Ellington

My homework didn't go well, and I needed to work with Donna to complete it. I had to name synonyms for such words as big, strong, escape, package. My computer homework was easier. I had to describe things that made me happy. I recounted my sons' graduation from college, my 50th birthday party, seeing my son walk into my hospital room after my stroke, and having three good people to work with after my brain attack. I also described things that I really disliked (mopping the floor, housework, unloading groceries from the car, getting into a cold car in winter, and being unable to make money).

My son Scott called in the evening and told me that he had a big test in paramedic school. I am sure he will be a good paramedic. He has a caring heart.

February 16, 1999

No great thing is created suddenly.
Epictetus

I told Steve that my right ankle rolls over when I walk, and I asked him to give me some exercises to help me to change that.

I reached a milestone. My therapy with Debbie and Steve decreased to three days a week from five. Speech therapy will continue to be five days a week.

I'm amazed that it's easier to write in powder than on paper. When I write in powder, my finger seems to write by itself as if it knows what my mind wants to spell.

I am going to San Antonio with Jane and Michael to see my parents. Mom and Dad are paying for my plane ticket and giving a luncheon for the people in their village who have been praying for me. I will be gone almost a week.

FROM THE OCCUPATIONAL THERAPIST

I sensed Polly's need to have some kind of control in her life, so I let her decide what goals we would pursue. I respected and admired her desire to understand her deficits and the goal of her therapies . We have been working on math skills, telling time, and using money.

FROM THE PHYSICAL THERAPIST.

Polly reported that her right ankle rolls over (inversion), so I started her on towel toe curls. She repeatedly picks up a towel with her toes to strengthen her ankle.

February 17, 1999

Adopt the pace of nature.
Her secret is patience.
Ralph Waldo Emerson

When I was changing planes today, I felt as if I was traveling for business as I used to do. Driving from the airport in San Antonio, we stopped to pick up Mexican food for dinner. As soon as we got to my parents' house, we had a Mexican food feast. Boy, do I miss Mexican food!

February 19, 1999

Worry often gives a small thing a big shadow.
Swedish Proverb

I wanted to be able to spell again, and I didn't want people to trivialize my spelling problems by telling me to use spell check. It's good that my therapists won't be giving tests. When I think about it, though, all my days since the stroke have been tests. I don't worry about grades. I guess that the stroke stripped away layers of worry. I only have time to worry about speaking again. Rehabilitation takes stamina and a sense of purpose to complete.

Although I try not to think about it, the incident in Burlington is engraved on my soul. I replay in my mind the nurse's words when she said in a loud, forceful voice, "No. You just watch me." Several people have told me that the poor care in the ward where I stayed was an open secret in the medical center. If so many people knew about it, why didn't they do anything about it?

81

Brain Attack

February 20, 1999

There is a way out of every dark mist over a rainbow trail.

A Navajo song

Yesterday I wrote an e-mail to Donna asking if she would want to write an article with me. I wanted it to be like a diary from the perspectives of both client and therapist. She said we should go for it!

The luncheon that my parents gave for me was delightful, and it was a good way for me to practice conversational speaking.

Some of my Houston friends sent me a plane ticket so I can go see them. I'm not anxious about traveling alone to Houston. I'm excited to see all my friends, as I miss them so.

Every day in my war with words, I churned out practice. I hated when I sounded stupid when I talked. It might sound silly, but I wanted to remember how I sounded when I couldn't speak. It was the episode of "brank," the only word I could say after the stroke. One of my nurse friends asked me what "brank" was. When I looked puzzled, she told me that brank was the word I had been saying. I shook my head in dismay. I didn't have a clue what brank meant.

I learned how to express sympathy by working with parents who had lost a child. I had never lost a child to death, and I learned not to say inane things to grieving parents like, "I know how you feel." This was the same as when people said, "I know how you feel when you can't add and subtract." It rubbed the only nerve that I had left. Unless they had had a stroke, they didn't know!

I admitted to myself that I must say good-bye to my past life. What a jolt of sadness this triggered in me.

A.P. and Theda

I didn't get to see Paulina until she was well enough to travel to Texas. We had talked with her frequently, and she had progressed to making herself understood. If you listened patiently and helped her, she would try to say words. Some words she couldn't say, and she used other sounds for these words.

While she was visiting, she worked hard. I noticed that she was impatient and frustrated and didn't listen to reason at times. She couldn't understand numbers at all, so we played dominoes so that she could learn some math again. Her memory seemed to be good with other things.

February 21, 1999

One does not make friends, one recognizes them.

Irene Dunn

I flew to Houston and the airport was noisy and crowded, but I navigated through it by myself. Questions like, "*Where do I go first?*" kept coming into my mind. I kept checking everything just to be sure that I was doing all right. It was good that I'm a woman and don't mind asking questions. It must be terrible for men, who usually hate to ask directions. In the boarding lounge with many people around and kids running, screaming, and crying, I was able to write a journal entry despite the distractions.

I saw a lot of friends, and when we were together, we seemed to be the way we were before the stroke except that I couldn't talk very well. Their wanting to see me made me feel so cherished. I watched when they moved at lightning speed over their words. I labored over every sound, and that left me far behind in the conversation. Sometimes I just listened instead of talking.

February 22, 1999

Life is either a daring adventure or nothing.
Security does not exist in nature.

Helen Keller

I met with my friend Robin in San Antonio and tried to converse with her. This was the first time I talked to someone about work-related things. She was patient and didn't try to finish my sentences for me as some people do. I enjoyed the afternoon but talking took a lot out of me.

Donna sent me an e-mail at my folks' house with questions for me to answer about my trip. She apologized if that sounded like homework. I typed back that she had told me that I wouldn't have to do homework on the trip, so I would consider her questions a note among friends.

My dad gave me my grandmother's dominoes to practice my math with. It was a lovely present as I was close to my grandmother. She was a good role model for me. I am like her in many respects – determined and feisty.

Robin R.

I was excited to see Polly when she came to town to visit her parents. I wasn't bothered by her hesitations in speech while she searched for the words that matched her thoughts. Her speech was wobbly, but her mind was the same.

When our afternoon ended, she seemed appreciative of my confidence in her and my patience as she searched for words. I hadn't focused on her disability. Instead, I saw her strength and knew that she would one day be back in the obstetrics spotlight. I saw the glow in her eyes as she talked about obstetrics-related things.

February 23, 1999

The doors of wisdom are never shut.
Benjamin Franklin

I struck up a conversation with a woman on the airplane back to Vermont, and she said that her secretary had just suffered a stroke. I promised to send her information about stroke treatments and therapies.

February 24, 1999

When life deals you lemons, make a pie.

I told Steve that my right thigh hurt, and I concluded that the nerves were regenerating. The pain didn't bother me. If I could give birth to a baby without drugs, this should be a piece of cake.

I watched Donna when she talked. She talked with little effort. Consonants and vowels rolled from her mouth like a waterfall. I wondered if I would ever talk like that again.

FROM THE PHYSICAL THERAPIST.

Polly seems to be happier since she returned from her vacation. She worked on the Nu-step for 23 minutes and marched in place on the trampoline with her eyes closed (balancing is harder with the eyes closed than with them open). I can see her strength coming back at every session.

Polly reported that she has more feeling in her leg. Her right thigh hurts. I explained that pain often accompanies the return of sensation.

FROM THE OCCUPATIONAL THERAPIST

I was so excited for Polly when she returned from her trip to Texas. She had some difficulty with distracting environments, but she was fully functional in busy airports when trying to find her gates.

February 25, 1999

What lies behind us and what lies before us
are small matters compared to what lies within us.
Ralph Waldo Emerson

I can do most things by myself, and I plan to get better through sheer willpower, endurance, and grit. But some days are harder than others. Today I tried to say something, but the words mingled together and came out as a mish-mash of sounds. I need Donna to give me direction when I lose my bearings. She remarked that I look different, because I am more animated in my speech. I hadn't realized that since the stroke, I lost enjoyment in small things. The trip to Texas restored that pleasure.

My leg hurt especially at night, but feeling pain was better than feeling nothing. The only thing that helped was sitting in a hot bath. I was getting a dose of my own medicine. When my labor clients complained about their pain, I told them that pain was good. They would love to see me now.

Sometimes it was tough to have faith in the rehab process. I told Eric, "Please don't make me do any more." But I did do more, because what else could I do except keep going on? I told myself to suck it up and go wearily on.

Dee

Correspondence was a healthy outlet for Polly's worries about her career, her loss of income, and her dependence on others. She recognized that depression was to be expected, and she asked me to send cards that made her laugh. She needed my assurance that I would not abandon her.

Eric

I drove Polly to rehab every day, because it was what I could do to help her regain her career. I drove to my job every day, so I just drove to a hospital too.

Brain Attack

February 26, 1999

A friend is what the heart needs all the time.
Henry Van Dyke

It is two months since the stroke, and my schedule in rehab has decreased to three days a week even though the going is slow.

I feel as if I am sleepwalking through my life. I feel dull, and I grope in my wordless mind for anything spirited. I have to think so hard about everything, not only speaking. I used to be a spontaneous and animated person. I miss being able to carry on a conversation. I miss chatting with abandon. I don't take anything for granted anymore.

February 27, 1999

Words are the fuel for my hungry mind. Sometimes I feel that I am in a fantasy land of mirrors where everything is reversed. My words would return to normal if I could get out of this hall of mirrors.

I hate jarring sounds. They make my brain feel as if it was being sliced by a knife.

<u>Stephanie</u>

Polly thought and spoke slowly, but she still had the great mind that I so respected. She just needed longer to express herself. I had to work at finding the correct pace between talking so slowly that she was insulted and talking so fast that she couldn't understand me and became frustrated. Many times I knew what she was trying to say, but I didn't feel right finishing the thought for her. It seemed more respectful to give her the moment or two that she needed to prod her brain and come up with the right word.

It is a longstanding joke that when people talk to someone who speaks a foreign language, they tend to speak more loudly as if that will compel the person to understand them. With Polly, I had to fight the tendency to think that because her speech was slower, her mind must be slower too. Her mind was sharp. She seemed to have retained most of her knowledge; she simply needed more time to retrieve it. Yet when you hear someone speaking that slowly and deliberately, the natural tendency is to begin to speak to her as if she is mentally slow.

February 28, 1999

You are here.

I watched people talk. Maybe I thought that I would get better by osmosis.

I had trouble pulling words apart into their constituent sounds called phonemes. What an odd word that seemed to me. I learned from Donna that English has 40 phonemes, the smallest discernible segments of speech.

One of my friends visited and asked if I wanted help when I was searching for a word. The nicest thing was that she asked. I don't like people to speak for me unless absolutely necessary. But sometimes it is just too hard, and I let them complete the word or phrase. My friend told me that I am an inspiration to her. I carry those words in my heart.

I put away the powder that I was using to spell. I was on a roll with the writing stuff. I wish that the talking stuff was better.

I can't hold numbers in my mind long enough to dial a telephone, and that makes me feel stupid.

The beautiful potted plant from a friend in Phoenix gave me was still blooming. I thought about her every day when I saw it. It was amazing that that kind of thing helped me so much.

Two weeks ago I found a magazine ad that looked like how my life feels. It showed a figure climbing a mountain. The caption read, "You are here." The ad was for an Outward Bound program and asked, "Which do you conquer first?" The answer, the ad implied, was fear. That was wrong. In all this time, I wasn't fearful, but other feelings did surface including sadness, anger, tiredness, wonderment, thankfulness, frustration, gladness, awe, and peace. Like the climber in the ad, I wondered how this would turn out. My plans for my future were in flux.

As I got better, I found a new respect for my brain.

Chapter Seven
Soul Searching

March 1, 1999

Happiness is not something you experience;
it is something you remember.

Oscar Levant

When Eric was at work, I felt like a prisoner, because I couldn't go anywhere by myself.

I had a conversation with Donna today about not working as a public speaker again until I could give my audiences their money's worth. I was at the top of my game when the stroke happened, and I won't give people less than that. I have to think more about the people I would be talking to than about myself. I felt overwhelmed with decisions about my professional future.

I needed to face the fact that the recovery process was slow. That was hard for a woman like me who lived life at full tilt.

I am still holding back a little in my relationship with Donna until I can decide if I can trust her with my emotions and my whole being. This hesitation is part of the legacy from my experience in the medical center. I still remember how it felt when the nurses betrayed me. Will I be safe?

I worked on syllables again to help me say words better. Donna told me that when I needed to say a word, I should visualize the first letter. I put my mouth in gear for the first letter only and then finished the word. When I thought about what word to write or say, I saw it like a theater in my mind.

I worked on what Donna called "chunking," a technique that could help me remember lists and numbers. I would chunk the numbers into groups of twos at first. Eventually I would be able to remember bigger chunks.

If I had trouble when I was typing, I wrote the word in long hand first. It seemed that my brain sent my hand a message about the correct letter.

I worked on what others told me to do, and I felt as if others were running my life, but I really couldn't run my life right now. The stroke made me impotent.

FROM THE OCCUPATIONAL THERAPIST

Polly needed to talk and express her feelings. I talked with her about her life and profession so that I could get to know her better. It helped me to guide her therapy toward meaningful goals.

Polly would exhaust herself at home. Therapy was her new career, and she made it a full-time job. Polly's attitude and perseverance put my life into perspective. She always inspired me with her get-it-done attitude.

March 3, 1999

Decisions, Decisions

I entered a dark hole when I lost my speech, and sometimes I didn't think I would get out of it. Some days, I felt like a yo-yo, alternating between optimism and despair. Today was one of the despairing days, as I had to cancel a summer speaking engagement. When I told the conference organizers to get a substitute, I felt better – as if a large weight had been taken off my shoulders. I knew that more engagements would have to be canceled before I was through.

I slept only four hours last night. I felt that my professional life was going down the drain. I did print some labor-support cards [information for people who help women during labor] on the computer, so I could help Eric keep our publishing business afloat. I thought about how my education was not being used. Sometimes I felt that I was watching from above the room and could see myself doing things that looked stupid. Was this someone's life? Was this what my life had become?

On the other hand, I finished two pages of idioms, and I realized that I couldn't have done them two weeks before. I tried to pronounce all the words on the pages, while before I couldn't have even remembered what to do. A single-minded focus helped me forge ahead.

Keep your face to the sunshine, and you cannot see the shadow.
Helen Keller

I missed having my Houston friends to lean on, and not having them nearby made my recovery more difficult. I was thankful that I would be able to see them later in the month.

I could tell that people whom I talked to on the phone wanted to end the conversation as soon as they could because it took me so long to say anything. Sometimes I wanted to explain my situation to them, but I decided that the explanation wasn't worth the effort needed to say the words.

I needed to accept that my past life was over, and I needed to lower my expectations for my life. I had so much knowledge in my brain, but I couldn't get the information out. What a loss of an education.

I had to keep calm so I wouldn't break down. I wished I could speak again as I used to, but that wasn't going to happen. Speaking was a lost dream.

Therapy was so important to me, but in the back of my mind lurked the fear of being unable to continue with it because of financial concerns. Eric said not to worry about it, but I did.

FROM THE PHYSICAL THERAPIST.

Polly's gait is improving, and she lurches forward less when she walks. Polly was ready to decrease the frequency of her PT sessions.

Polly's speech is better, but several times I had no idea what she was trying to say. For most stroke patients, the most important thing is walking better. I never had the feeling that walking was Polly's top priority. I asked her if she wouldn't care about walking if she could speak well. She responded, "I wouldn't be bothered if I couldn't walk if I could talk."

March 4, 1999

Plunge boldly into the thick of life.

Goethe

It dawned on me that I had been suspended in the rehab effort while waiting for my life to begin again. But it wouldn't begin again; this was my life. The act of writing my diary gave my life the depth and intimacy that was missing from it without speech.

I felt better, and I seemed to be speaking a little better. Although speaking still demanded great effort, I didn't have to grope so hard to think of words, and my writing seemed better too. My life was a roller coaster of emotions. I would feel really bad, and then when it seemed my brain was reconnecting a little better, I would feel good again.

In the afternoon, I felt myself fading. When I couldn't talk or read because my brain seemed on overload, I stared out the window and watched the snow fall in my newly adopted state. I was grateful that I could see more from the window in Vermont than I could in the crowded subdivision in Texas where I used to live. There the only view was one stately magnolia tree in my yard.

I pondered what my path in life was and what my enforced sabbatical meant. Perhaps I was focusing on the pebbles under my feet and not on where my feet were going.

March 5, 1999

We can no longer afford to throw away even an 'unimportant'
day by not noticing the wonder of it all.
We have to be willing to discover and then appreciate
the authentic moments available to all of us every day.
Sarah Ban Breathnach

Donna gave me homework to do on the computer. She told me that she was giving me food for thought. I had to describe peanut butter with as many adjectives as I could. She asked me to describe to someone what it was like have regained my ability to read and write.

My exhaustion was bone deep, and I never felt so tired before in my life.

March 6, 1999

If somebody believes in you,
and you believe in your dreams, it can happen.
Tiffany Bangs

I thought about my rehab team and why so few teams worked as well as mine did. I decided that success depended on the power of the relationships among the team members and on their developing an emotional bond. My therapists seemed to have genuine feelings for each other. They communicated confidence to each other, and it spilled over to me. They shared in my successes. Their good natures won my confidence. My team drew me in, motivated me, made me feel special, and made a difference in my life. The healing relationship developed over time. I had done a good job of surrounding myself with those people, and I hoped I could teach something to them about the power of determination and perseverance.

March 7, 1999

Patience is a by-product of tribulations.

I felt like my old self today. That was a hopeful sign. I kept telling myself that I was unstoppable and I couldn't let this stroke get me down, but that was easier said than done. I was learning about things that I didn't really want to know, but education might be the way out of the quagmire I was in.

Was this episode what life was about? Was the lesson finished? Was this episode a rite of passage?

FROM THE SPEECH THERAPIST

Polly was speaking in phrases, writing sentences, reading sentences, and beginning to work on everyday math. Polly went right out to the store, bought first-grade math workbooks, and started her way up the ladder to relearn math facts. The occupational therapist and I gave her strategies to help herself with money and time in everyday situations. The strategies included buying things with a credit card when she could so she wouldn't have to count out money, using a calculator, and not trying to give exact change for a purchase.

March 8, 1999

People have to drive me everywhere. I'm thankful they help, but I feel like a burden and I don't like that. People who know me seem accustomed to my dysfunction, but I'm not. I want to be more like I used to be.

I spent two hours talking with Debbie and Donna. Donna said I was speaking better, but I still felt like I was in deep and hazardous water when I spoke. Otherwise, I felt more like my old self. I sent a long e-mail about obstetrics-related topics to a colleague. That was the first time that I wrote about clinical things.

Donna broke her wrist. I told her that I couldn't speak, and she couldn't write, and together we might be one whole person.

I thought about how people react when they realize something is wrong with me. Their faces are a mixture of emotions–fright, worry, dread, anxiety, distress, solicitude, care, and concern. I want to tell them to put themselves in my shoes, but it reminds them too much that "except by God's grace there go I."

93

March 9, 1999

*You try to make an interesting journey between
the cradle and the grave, you know.*
Robert Duvall

As I tried to say more words, it still helped me to see Donna say them – the trick I first used in the hospital. I wanted to jump like an athlete over the hurdles that separated me from my words. It was fortunate that Donna's education was in speech, language, and psychology because my feelings and my inability to speak affected each other.

I try to treasure this experience and the accompanying grief because I know that I will learn from them, but this outlook is hard sometimes. My past life is receding. Now I have a life of mispronounced words.

March 11, 1999

When love and skill work together, expect a masterpiece.
John Ruskin

I slept a long time at night and awoke feeling lousy. Like an old woman, I still get up stiffly from sitting or lying down. I try to recall the saying "you can cry because roses have thorns or celebrate that thorns have roses," but sometimes that's hard to remember.

I had to cancel another of my speaking engagements, and it seems hopeless to think that I could make a living as a public speaker. This loss of language sucks!

March 12, 1999

Boldness has genius, power, and magic in it.
Goethe

Today I felt better, and when I started talking, the words came out right. I felt that my brain was reconnecting. It was nice to use words with less difficulty.

Donna used another innovative learning strategy with me. Since I could distinguish sounds better, she taught me to divide words into syllables by using wooden blocks to represent the syllables. I would say the syllable each block represented and then put the blocks – and syllables – together to make a word and say it.

People ask me if I'm depressed, but I haven't been. I have been angry and frustrated, but I will not let this stroke ruin my life.

As Donna's wrist was bothering her, I found that I was being a caretaker, a role that was so familiar to me. It was nice to feel less dependent.

March 13, 1999

Let the world know you as you are,
not as you think you should be.
Fanny Brice

I felt blah, as if I was seeing life though a cloudy mirror. Once again, I begged my brain to release my voice. I didn't want to imagine a world without words, and I was sucked into a vortex of emotions once again.

When one of my friends read part of the journal that I'm writing, she said she was shocked at my doubts because it had not crossed her mind that I would not get back to normal and resume my career. Doubts about my future cross my mind a lot these days. Will I have a career ever again?

I worked on exercises that made me shift my perspective when I described things. I had to describe a table for example. What is it? Hard, soft, made of wood. Who uses it? Families. What do you do with it? Eat on it. Set things on it. I had a lot of trouble describing things. I knew what a table was, but I couldn't tell you. The exercise helped.

Maureen

Polly's speaking is improved, but mornings are still better for her. She has trouble speaking at night as she is tired from her therapies, but we always have some laughs no matter how tired she is.

March 14, 1999

People who believe a problem can be solved
tend to get busy solving it.
William Raspberry

I finished my fourth-grade multiplication book. Sometimes when I'm working on a child's arithmetic book, I feel foolish but not enough to stop working. The numbers don't seem so foreign to me now. I came this far on sheer will, and now nothing will stand in my way.

Donna lent me a game to help me both read and write. It has words on cards, and I group the words into sentences. Once that would have been so easy.

The e-mails that people send me tell me how strong I am. I carry this image around with me every day.

I didn't expect to be able to say a word perfectly, but I wanted to be able to get at least close to perfect. Sometimes I could, but other times my attempts were dismal failures.

Seeing the report that the insurance company needed to let me keep going in rehab was an eye-opening experience. Damn, I was severely injured by the stroke. I had never seen so many huge words in my life, and they all described my deficits. Looking at the diagnoses had the opposite effect on me than it would have had on most people. It convinced me that I could get better. But then I've never been like most people.

March 15, 1999

With ordinary talents and extraordinary perseverance
all things are attainable.

Thomas Buxton

I was practicing words that have blends-letters that are said in different parts of the mouth. You say p, b, v, t, and d with your lips; sh, s, and z with your mouth; and k and g with your throat. So I said words like strict and thrust to make me change how I made the sounds.

As far as my emotions were concerned, I still felt that storm clouds hovered over my head, and then the hugest rainstorm would hit and I would cry and cry. Sometimes I cried for a reason, but other times I didn't know why I was crying.

My life seems like a story that you read voraciously to see what happens next. I thought about this episode in my life and tried to be hopeful. My life stretches ahead of me, and I know that I am the person shaping it.

I may be finished with OT next week – another milestone. I talked with Debbie about how I felt when my brain seemed to be reconnecting. Saturday was one of the days when I felt really lousy. I couldn't talk as well as I usually did, and I slept more. I realized that on the day after a bad day, I would usually discover that I had made progress in some way. It was as if my brain was working hard on something and couldn't do anything else. I decided not to do anything when my brain was switching gears. It was fascinating how my brain was working.

Eric

I never treated Polly any differently after the attack than I did before so she would gain confidence that she would be all right. Many people treated her as if she couldn't function as before and tried to do everything for her, including finishing her sentences. Our boys and I knew Polly as well as anyone could, and we knew that eventually she would be back to her old self. The boys felt that anyone who thought differently didn't know how determined Polly could be. They had been on the receiving end of her you-can-do-it attitude. They learned the hard way not to argue with their mother unless they had all their facts because she would always call their bluff. Polly always told them that they could do anything they wanted if they worked hard, and they knew she was doing that too.

Polly had a tendency to look at me when she was talking to others, and I had to remind her to look at them instead of at me.

March 17, 1999

Do what you can, with what you have, where you are.
Theodore Roosevelt

I went to Houston again, and Eric and I hit the ground running. Some of our friends hadn't seen me since the stroke. Much as I enjoyed the visits, the frantic pace from dawn to dark was hard for me.

We went to dinner with our friends Peter and Nancy and had a marvelous time.

Peter

My wife, Nancy, and I went out to dinner with Polly and unknowingly chose a restaurant that had an oral menu. This would be a challenge for anyone, but it was impossible for Polly. I noticed that she had significant muscle weakness on her right side, but her biggest problems were recognizing words and speaking.

By the end of the evening, though, her speech reminded me of that of a foreigner who needed practice in English conversation. She would misspeak or mispronounce words, but overall her speech was rather charming. When she expressed apprehension over being capable of speaking to groups again, I suggested that she warn her audiences that she was relearning the English language.

Brain Attack

Nancy

At dinner Polly relied on Eric's help. If she was struggling to recall words, Eric came to her rescue. Many polysyllabic words were too difficult for her to say. She would frequently mix up the order of her sentences, but she was determined to speak, and only occasionally did she get frustrated. She spoke of periodically having very difficult days followed by good days. She laughed when I suggested that, like a computer, she needed to download on occasion.

March 25 1999

It is not a matter of thinking much but also loving much
So do whatever most kindles love in you.
Mother Teresa

In my PT session, I accused Steve of trying to kill me as the exercises were more difficult. I hope harder exercises mean that I'm getting better.

My occupational therapist asked me to help her give birth to her baby later in the year. It was so nice of her to want my help. She didn't care whether my speech was perfect.

I don't have to search so hard for words anymore when I write, but I still alternate between optimism and despair. It has been three months since the stroke, and though my recovery is going well, it's slower than I want. When I can't believe in myself, I trust that Eric, Donna, and others were right when they said that I will be able to resume my career. It's okay to hope.

March 26, 1999

Downloading Days

Today was what my Houston friend Nancy called a downloading day. I didn't feel right, but I managed to take an order on the phone by myself because Eric wasn't there. I even got the credit card numbers right. The customer was patient as I wrote down all the numbers. Ta da!

I continued the voice and breathing exercises that Donna gave me. I had to match the volume and timing of loud and soft sounds with my breathing. I had to sing a descending scale of four or five notes with the sounds, mmmmm, vvvvv, and zzzzz. I was sounding like a bee and a car. It was good that no one was home except Eric; people would have thought that I had lost my mind. I could hear the comments: "I used to know Polly when she could talk, and now all she does is make buzzing noises."

Through e-mail, Donna told me, "I still can't believe your writing. It is so very fluent and you 'sound' really good." A few of the words I wrote during the day included inundated, managed, discharged, and biopsychosocial. And I didn't use spell check! I hoard my new words like the treasures that they are.

I got a letter from a friend in Houston and made Eric listen to me read the whole thing. The poor guy will be glad when I quit telling him, "Listen to me." In an "aha!" moment, I remembered the first whole sentence that I could say, "Come here quick," so I'm still in the same vein of giving Eric orders.

Two friends are coming to dinner tomorrow night, and I'll have someone else to talk to. It might give Eric a rest!

March 27, 1999

Strange Buzzing Noises

In an e-mail congratulating me on my hard work, a friend asked, "does this mean you might be ready for a conference in October?" She said that she wouldn't mind if I was making buzzing sounds. She would name the session: "Buzz Session with Polly Perez!" It was gratifying to be wanted, but I still had reservations about doing a good job as a public speaker.

I finished a cross-stitch piece that I had been working on for a month or two. It was a quote from Swindell: "We are all faced with a series of great opportunities, brilliantly disguised as impossible situations." It was for Donna's office. I wanted it to help empower people who were learning to speak again.

FROM THE SPEECH PATHOLOGIST

Polly did not take the time to consider that she would not recover. Her husband, Eric, having been married to Polly for more than 30 years, agreed. Nevertheless, there were many ups and downs and days when Polly had doubts. The plaque that she embroidered for me said it all.

March 28, 1999

By your endurance, you will gain your lives.
Luke 21:19

Friends came for dinner, and I couldn't talk to them. I slept in the afternoon, but the nap didn't help me. Usually I had no one to talk to, and then people were here and I couldn't talk at all. Speaking seemed to take more effort than it was worth. I explained things simply because elaborating was too much trouble. The dinner was frustrating and exasperating, but I wouldn't let it get me down.

I miss the joy that I used to have in words, which shaped my life, but Donna helped me focus on my strengths and reminded me not to be so hard on myself. I have always been my hardest critic. Donna celebrates my accomplishments just as I do.

My leg has more feeling in it.

March 29, 1999

The greatest pleasure in life is doing what people say you cannot do.
Walter Bagehot

I did 11 pages of homework that included volume exercises. I made the sound of the sea, ebbing and flowing. I started softly, increased the sound, and then finished softly again. It was really good that no one was with me. I was sure that I looked like an idiot making weird faces, but I did it because Donna thought it would help me.

Eric is leaving for two days to work in the lower part of the state. I will stay with Jane and Michael, and they'll take me to rehab. They have been so good to me, and I knew that my schedule is hard for them.

I was working on giving a two-day seminar in Ohio on labor support. Donna told me that was not a crazy thing to do. Part of me wanted to say no to the request, but another part told me I should do it. I was raised with a strong work ethic, and it sometimes gets me into trouble by making me say yes when I should say no.

I found out that my physical therapy might be done in a couple of weeks. My right leg feels more like part of my body – almost normal.

I keep thinking about what the lesson of the stroke was. I haven't figured it out. Maybe it wasn't a lesson, just bad luck.

March 30, 1999

To endure what is unendurable is true endurance.
Japanese Proverb

I can communicate on paper better than I can talk. In my mind, I plan the words I want to say. I crave my former relationship to spoken words.

I read that the brain consumes 25 per cent of the body's energy production. No wonder I'm tired! My little grey brain cells are working overtime. Fatigue from thinking all day was overwhelming. Tiredness dragged me down to sleep again.

Donna told me that I would have special blessings at the end of this journey. My speech, occupational, and physical therapists were one of the special blessings that she was referring to. I knew that I was the person who had to do the work of getting better, but it surely helped to have people like them in my corner.

March 31, 1999

Learning is a treasure that will follow its owner everywhere.
Chinese Proverb

In my mind I could generate ideas to write about, but I still groped for words to explain the ideas. I cherished the part of myself that could explain things. I wished that I could say enough to tell people how I felt about complex subjects. The paucity of language made me sad.

FROM THE SPEECH PATHOLOGIST

Polly's comprehension and speech were noticeably faster. We continued to work on phonology. She used wooden blocks to help her segment sounds and syllables into words and phrases. The tactile component helped decrease her apraxia.

FROM THE PHYSICAL THERAPIST

Polly appears ready to be weaned from PT.

Chapter Eight
Ambitious Goals

April 1, 1999

Courage is the price that life exacts for granting peace.
Amelia Earhart

When I was writing, the words seemed to flow better and faster from my mind, but my speech was still impoverished.

I could feel more of my face, legs, and hands, and I welcomed the accompanying pain that signaled that was I getting better.

My ambition transcends simply being able to speak again. I want to go back to my profession of public speaking. Some days the process of recovery was hell, and I told myself that it was better than being dead, but when I was at my lowest ebb, I didn't believe that. Some days, I couldn't say anything right. Speaking was still laborious, arduous, and formidable, and it was endurable only because Donna made the task of speaking doable and desirable. Even though she helped me, I sometimes felt as if my words were melting down.

I was dancing as fast as I could to remake my shattered life. Now my life seemed like a stiff waltz, but I wanted to fox trot or jitterbug. I reminded myself that patience is a virtue. I recalled that on the second day after the brain attack, Marje hung a poster in my hospital room that said, "Patience."

FROM THE PHYSICAL THERAPIST

Polly told me that she was confident in her physical abilities, and her biggest concern was her speech.

April 3, 1999

Ever want to scream?

Sometimes I pretended that nothing in my life had changed. Then I had to talk. Today I felt hopelessly inept. I couldn't speak very well in the morning even though I was bursting at the seams with the words that I wanted to say. When something like that happened, I would think that I couldn't work anymore. How would I be able to speak publicly again if I couldn't even say what was on my mind?

When I gave up trying to explain what I wanted to say, deep sobs erupted and I raged all the way up the stairs crying, "I hate this!" I had never felt so utterly beaten. I cried so much that I thought that my head would blow up.

April 4, 1999

Out of sync.

It was another day of exhaustion. I was out of step. This was unrelenting warfare, and I was battling for control of my words. At times the battle was comical–the words that came out of my mouth were not what I wanted to say.

I used to talk so easily, and now my speech was halting part of the time. I felt like a caged bird that could remember being free. Someday I will fly again. Then just watch me soar. Failure is not an option.

I craved words of praise, and this was new for me. I didn't usually seek others' approval. Most of my life I had found the will to achieve inside of me, and I didn't like asking for compliments. Now I often asked, "Am I doing good?".

FROM THE SPEECH PATHOLOGIST

I proposed to Polly that we use the text of some of her previous speeches in therapy. Polly was already writing on her computer. She was using the telephone with greater ease, and her words were flowing more smoothly. We were at about the "three-syllable-word stage" in fluency. When Polly was able to both visualize words and see them in print, her fluency increased. So there we were in high school English and speech class 101. Vocabulary exercises: synonyms, antonyms, homonyms, figurative language, and metaphor. Polly started writing with a vengeance. "I'm going to write a book...this needs to be told...what it's like...for others to understand," she said. She was absolutely correct. I had other stroke clients who needed to hear Polly and to speak with her. She was already becoming a powerful advocate not only for herself, but also for others. About four months post-stroke, we decided that Polly should write a speech and present it to others in the Rehab Department.

April 5, 1999

The Birth of a Book

The more that I thought about it, the more I realized that the article about my stroke needed to be a book instead. The words that I had written meant a lot to me. I was pleased that I could spell, and that my writing was going well. Being able to write was freedom and power. My life had very little of either. I had completed 32 pages. It helped me to know that I could still do something well.

I worried about the medical bills that we couldn't afford to pay. I was usually the one who managed our finances, and I couldn't do it. I found an ad that reflected how I felt. It showed a patient wearing a hospital gown. He had an IV line in his arm, and he was standing in front of a huge stack of dirty dishes, washing them. A sign said, "This is your hospital; please help keep it clean." The caption read, "How do you plan on paying unexpected medical bills?" I knew how the guy felt.

I haven't talked well for three days. I shouldn't even think about working as a public speaker. I wanted to quit trying, but something inside me wouldn't let me. I talked to one of my doctors about my feeling lousy for three days. I found that I felt better at night. He didn't have an explanation for me. I guess I will have to figure it out myself.

Four months after the brain attack, I had bad dreams about the nurse who told me, "No. You just watch me." I could hear the tone in her voice and see the look in her eyes. I felt like my clients who had post-traumatic stress disorder. Perhaps I had it too.

To help me articulate, I said pairs of words containing the same sounds. I did better with words that started differently, such as fight-bite, vote-boat, fall-mall, than with words that ended differently, as in tub-tough, seep-seethe, and robe-rove. I still didn't like having much background noise if I needed to concentrate a lot. I was impatient for more periods of animation and creativity as my life is filled with sameness.

My birthday has always been special, but I couldn't get excited about this one. Someone asked me what I wanted for my birthday, and I replied that all I wanted was my speech back.

<u>Julie</u>

Through Polly's e-mails I watched her burrow her way out of her affliction. With each note, her postings got longer and more complex.

April 6, 1999

Seeds of faith are always within us;
Sometime it takes a crisis to nourish their growth.

Susan L Taylor

Today I was throwing words around the room. I would say parts of a sentence and try to propel the words into different places in the room, as Donna taught me. I tried to enunciate and speak slowly. The exercise helped me project the words as well as say them correctly. It also helped me feel strong instead of weak and dejected.

One of my friends sent me a message that she was proud of the work I was doing to get well. She wrote that stroke victims need my kind of loving support and no one could give that support better than someone who had lived through the agony of a brain attack. The hours I have spent working on regaining the speech I lost are astonishing. My friend didn't know how much her words helped me.

Another friend reminded me that the Chinese word for crisis is composed of two figures: danger and opportunity. Perhaps the greatest danger in a crisis is to fail to see the opportunity in it. I wondered what the opportunities were for me in this crisis. I don't feel that the stroke was a catastrophe, but it sure was a hindrance. If there was any magic in this dance of change, it was in learning about character and endurance.

April 7, 1999

Wisdom is a blending of body, mind, and soul
balanced with experience.

I was steadily making my way to recovery, and my level of commitment was high. I had been pushed before but never like this. I accomplished a feat when I drove alone for the first time. It was a short trip, only ten miles. I badly wanted to drive so I wouldn't be so dependent on others. I had driven the car with Eric as a passenger, so I wasn't too nervous about driving alone. Debbie had told me that I could take an adaptive driver's program, but I didn't think it was necessary. When I drove into rehab, I said aloud in the car, "I did it!"

I told a friend in Connecticut that I was going to write a book about stroke recovery. Her response was fantastic! I was getting so many messages telling me I must write this book that I started toward that goal.

I so wanted to write professionally again that when I read a magazine or paper, I copied the words that I wanted to write; otherwise, I might not remember them. I wrote the reminders on the postcard inserts that came in magazines. These little bits of paper could be found littering every room of my house. I guess I could call the effort word recycling.

Eric was away, and I answered the phone for our office even though I couldn't communicate very well. I made callers repeat things more than twice, but I took a few orders. I realized that people talk so fast when they give numbers. I told one man that he needed to speak more slowly. A woman asked me how to become a doula. After a while I told her I had a stroke four months before and couldn't quickly say some of the words I wanted to say but I would eventually say what I needed. The word that I stumbled on was "organization."

Steve told me today that next week will be my last PT session.

FROM THE SPEECH PATHOLOGIST

Polly's conversational speech was very different from her formal speech, written language, or reading aloud. In conversational speech, Polly became adept at substituting a shorter or easier word for another word that she perceived as being too difficult to say. When she read aloud, wrote, or lectured, substitution was not an option.

FROM THE PHYSICAL THERAPIST

I discussed with Polly my plan to discontinue PT, and she accepted it. Her agility is much improved.

A Focal Point

Today's speech session went well. When I was trying to say a word, I focused on seeing it in my mind. I asked Donna if I would ever be able to speak as I once did. She answered yes, and she told me that I spoke better when I was impassioned about the subject.

I was grieving over the loss of a project. I am scheduled to speak in Cincinnati next weekend about obstetrics. I wish that I could speak well enough to go, but one of my friends from New York will have to give my speeches for me.

A friend from California thought that I have a moving and heartwarming start to my book. I hope that it will shed light on what stroke victims have to endure in rehabilitation. She said that she never knew what people who had a stroke went through, but after reading part of my journal she understood. From what they see from the outside, most people are unaware of my torment. To appreciate that, they must talk to me or read my journal.

April 8, 1999

Thank you for believing in me before I believed in myself.
Kobi Yamado

Debbie asked what we were doing in my speech session today, because she heard a lot of laughter coming from our room. I feel more spirited and playful – more like my old self. The laughter was about mistakes I made in pronunciation. I really fractured words today.

Adding words to my vocabulary is so tedious. I have trouble flowing with this experience. I'm a dismal failure at flowing!

April 9, 1999

What is a friend? A single soul dwelling in two bodies.
Aristotle

Just as I labored to write this book, I will prevail in speaking publicly again. I reminded myself that a friend's husband couldn't do anything at all after his stroke and he had conquered a lot. I can do it too!

I was getting better at interweaving tasks, but I couldn't do several things at once the way I used to. I can answer the phone and talk to someone, but I can't type at the same time. Before the brain attack, I could have answered the phone, typed on the computer, talked to someone, and given detailed directions, all at the same time.

I used to embrace discussion, and I missed that. It was so hard to have discussions with several people that most of the time I didn't even try.

A friend took me out to lunch for my birthday that's coming up over the weekend. I don't have many friends in Vermont, and it was a sweet gesture. The birthday lunch with her made me feel like I was back with my friends in Houston.

Jamie

Polly's speech was slow, as if she were choosing her words carefully, but her voice sounded like her, with the proper timbre and inflection--not the monotone she'd had earlier.

April 10, 1999

Do not fear or be dismayed.
Deuteronomy 2:21

I found an unorthodox way to improve my balance. I told Steve that I had been trying to walk toe to toe on the treadmill and had walked about a quarter mile. I tried harder things without being told because that's my style. Steve laughed, as he is used to my gung-ho attitude. My leg cramped at night again, and the only thing that made it better was soaking in hot water. The pain is still part of the nerves' healing.

My collateral circulation is improving. My toes have more feeling in them, although I still can't feel the middle of the palm of my hand.

I read a whole magazine story aloud in the way I want to be able to read aloud when I present a speech. But by 9:30 pm, I was tired of reading and concentrating, and I couldn't pronounce a word. That set up a crying jag. You would think that I would know when to stop reading.

I was so tired of everything. My recovery was so nerve-wracking. I was tired of being frustrated. I was so tired of being tired I could have cried, and I did. I felt trapped in a vicious cycle, and the day ended with a torrent of tears. I never have cried so much in my whole life as in the past four months. I would like my life to be normal again – whatever that means.

Enough whining...

April 12, 1999

You must be the change you wish to see in the world.
Mahatma Gandhi

I have thought many times since I had the stroke how important it is when you're hospitalized to have someone to act as your advocate, especially if you're aphasic. I was lucky that I had a sister-in-law who was a nurse and was so focused on me. But all patients deserve an advocate. Stroke care should be family-centered – a new way for patients and their families and health-care providers to relate to one another. Family-centered care is collaborative, and it promotes the full participation by patients and their families in the planning, delivery, and evaluation of health care. The family-centered stroke care philosophy recognizes that families and friends play a vital role in ensuring patients' health and well-being (see Appendex)

For the first time since the brain attack, I dreamed about birth and speaking publicly. In the dream, I could speak perfectly.

Today was a good day, and my speech session went well. I worked on saying these words:

unavoidable	Singapore	authorities	academic
poetry	affectionately	indiscriminately	

My writing was faster, and my reading aloud was a little better too, but speech was still a tough nut to crack. I used to have fun with words, and I collected words whose sound and meaning I liked, such as "iatrogenic." Iatrogenic sounds like a wonderful thing, but it means that something detrimental was mistakenly done in the hospital. Now words are not fun.

April 13, 1999

Courage is resistance to fear, mastery of fear,
not absence of fear.

Mark Twain

I had a good talking day. A friend who lived in Houston called, and we talked for about 30 minutes. She told me that I was talking faster.

A doula friend called to ask me to speak about communicating with nurses at a training session for doulas next month in Burlington, and I agreed. I talked to her for 30 minutes or so, and I didn't stumble over many words. The talk will be my first time speaking publicly. There is always a first time for everything, I told myself. For some reason, I didn't fear the speech. The worst thing that could happen was that I couldn't talk at all, but I didn't think that would happen.

A friend in Florida wants me to speak at a conference in late October, and we had a spirited conversation for about an hour. I was amazed that after hearing me speak, she still wanted me to give the talk. I told her that I had to think about it before I could give her an answer. I had many reservations. Was it too early for me to give a keynote address? Is that more than I can handle?

April 14, 1999

*The ultimate measure of a man
is not where he stands in moments of comfort, but where he
stands in times of challenge and controversy.*
Martin Luther King, Jr.

I got up early and worked on tongue twisters and difficult consonant clusters before I went to speech therapy. When I made myself speak louder, I felt stronger and more in control.

The role of a speech therapist is multi-faceted. Sometimes Donna told me not to be so hard on myself and to rest a little. Sometimes she needed to give me a pep talk. Sometimes she encouraged me to push a bit harder. When I could no longer be energetic about speaking, she reminded me to chill out.

April 15, 1999

*Light one candle instead of cursing the darkness
and pray for the wherewithal to sustain the flame.*
Eleanor Roosevelt

Sometimes when I said a word, it sounded foreign, and I had to say it a few times until it sounded right in my ears. Even if I said the word correctly the first time, I had to hear it often enough for the sound to sink into my brain.

My friend from Florida called to ask me again to speak in the Fall. I was uncomfortable saying "no," but I refused the invitation.

April 16, 1999

It is always possible to approach a goal by a detour.
Theodor Riek

When I completed my physical therapy rehabilitation, I felt like a champion. That was another hurdle that I had cleared since the first of December. I had had enough challenges to last a lifetime. Steve was a good therapist because he saw me as an individual. For a long time, the only time I would laugh was during my physical therapy sessions with him. Having a stroke is so serious, but Steve used humor to put a different spin on therapy. His jokes made it fun to do repetitive exercises.

Sometimes I wish that I could pluck a word out of the air and say it. I can't, but it's a good thought anyway.

FROM THE PHYSICAL THERAPIST

Today Polly was discharged from PT. I learned a lot working with her. She was always willing to look at things in another way to see whether something would work for her. Some people are naturally stubborn, but Polly was stubborn for a purpose. She always had a goal in mind.

FROM THE OCCUPATIONAL THERAPIST

Polly never lost her nursing skills or her intuitiveness. She knew that I was pregnant before I had the chance to tell her.

In OT Polly regained approximately 90 percent of the sensation and proprioception (awareness of where her body was in space) in her right arm and 100 percent of the fine motor control of her right hand. She relearned numbers well enough to tell time and count coins and bills. She learned to take phone calls and write down numbers while taking credit card orders in the Perez home business. She was driving again, which bolstered her sense of independence.

April 17, 1999

Never, never, ever give up.
Winston Churchill

I got up at 5:30 am, even though it was Saturday. I was disciplined enough to practice what Donna had given me. It took me an hour and a half.

Before the stroke I had agreed to give a speech at a conference of the Association for Women's Health, Obstetrical, and Neonatal Nursing (AWHONN) in Chicago in July. I realized that if I was going to give the speech I needed to work on it or get someone else to do it. I spent the day rewriting a speech I'd already written and decided to ask Donna on Monday about giving it.

My hyacinths and daffodils were popping up and had buds. I sat watching the birds play in the trees outside my window.

I talked to a friend on the phone for about an hour, but I made so many mistakes. The words that I could say yesterday were lost. Where had they gone? This frustrated me so. When I couldn't even hold a conversation on the phone, how would I speak to a group? At that very moment, I didn't think that giving a speech was a viable option. When I don't think that I can do something, I need to know that people believe in me and I need to set shorter-term goals.

At night I talked to a doctor friend from Boston for about an hour. I worked with her when she had her children. Even though it was late, I didn't make many mistakes. That was good, but why couldn't I talk better earlier in the day? Usually I had more problems later at night.

April 18, 1999

Hope is a waking dream.

Aristotle

I was determined to turn the miscue in my life into something positive. I walked for a hour on the treadmill in the morning, and I also walked outside.

I still have trouble with word retrieval. I can't seem to free the words in my mind from their hiding places.

For as long as I can remember, I had a love affair with the written word, and reading was one of my passions too. I was working on speaking with passion once again. One day, I would open my mouth wide and let the passion out.

FROM THE SPEECH PATHOLOGIST

I told Polly not to despair when she wasn't fluent and to think instead about how often she was fluent. Her difficulty stands out because she is fluent most of the time. I reminded her to work with the blocks and to tap out the sounds that she couldn't say. She was having trouble with the word "individual," for example, so I told her to make each block a syllable. In/ di/ vi/ du/ al would use five blocks. Then she could put them together to make the whole word. Another strategy was to tap her finger as she said each syllable.

An e-card from Mark and Jamie said, "Because you're not afraid to face the music, you find yourself leading the band." I guess that for the past four months I was able to face the music even when I didn't like the song.

I pointed out to myself that I could read while Eric was watching the TV, even though four months ago that was impossible. That was progress, and that kind of self-talk helped me. The mental pep talk was a trick I used to use when I was running, and I found that it helped me to stay motivated.

Sometimes I wanted so badly to say a word that I could taste it. I was trying to say hard words, and I practiced reading aloud – hard words, easy words, all for practice. When I reached my limit, I said to Eric, "Help me please make it better." My determination was tenacious most days, but by the end of the day my will would falter.

Eric

I knew that everything would work out, an attitude that was in my genes. My dad was the same way when my mother died. He had never cooked before, but he adapted well and told me, "What else could I do except learn to cook?" While Polly was relearning after the brain attack, I took what had been presented to me and tried to adapt to the situation. Polly was doing the same thing.

April 19, 1999

Valor is a gift. Those having it never know for sure whether they have it until the test comes.
Carl Sandburg

I worked out on the treadmill most days – three miles today.

I talked with Donna about my not speaking at large conferences for the rest of the year. I was still ambivalent about it. I thought I needed to take the rest of the year to get my body, mind, and spirit in shape, but I also felt pressure to get ready to speak at a large convention, and I worried about it.

I tried to pace myself so that I had some energy left at the end of the day, but the attempt was often a grim failure, and I went bed early and exhausted.

April 20, 1999

Tomorrow is another day.
Margaret Mitchell – Gone with the Wind

I told Donna that when I read a newspaper or magazine, I kept a list of words that I wanted to be able to use in conversation or writing. She said, "Only you would be doing your own therapy." She created a safe zone around me so that I could do the hard work of healing and speaking again. Words such as "your progress is amazing" helped sustain me when the going got rough.

Damn, this was hard. I had to write a letter to my friend in Florida to confirm that I couldn't speak at her convention. I didn't want to write it, but I had to. I wrote:"I talked with my speech therapist about your upcoming convention. I'm working hard to get my fluency back. She and I both thought that a lecture of the size of yours so soon was too much for me right now."

I felt that I was letting my friend down, but I had to give most of my energy to the rehab process so I could speak better sooner and return to the work

I love – motivating and teaching others.

I wished the conference was next year, as I might have been able to do it then, but I had to play the cards that I had been dealt.

I resisted the urge to call a friend, as I didn't want to bother her. But there was no one at my house, and I needed someone who understood how I felt and could tell me I would be all right. A hug might have helped.

Oh well, Polly, suck it up, I told myself. Quit whining. It could be worse.

In the afternoon, I did call my friend Ana. At the end of the conversation, she said, "You had most of the words in this conversation. I just listened." I could hear myself talking, and I didn't make mistakes. The rhythm of my words seemed right. It was the way I talked with friends before the stroke. This was another milestone. It would be nice if the progress would continue.

April 21, 1999

My strength lies solely in my tenacity.
Louis Pasteur

Although it was hard to turn down the convention in Florida, I needed to think of the refusal as letting go – in a positive sense – after which would come renewal and even greater strength, I hope.

A friend told me that when I felt bad and needed a helping hand, I should put one arm on the opposite shoulder and wrap the other arm around my body, and I would have an instant hug from her. That helped me, even though the hug was long distance.

I want my book to include my feelings because it is so important for health-care workers to pay attention to their patients' feelings and soul. In my book I was baring my soul to help others. The book was a little sliver of good in this calamity.

April 22, 1999

You don't get to choose how you're going to die and when.
You can only decide how you're going to live.
Joan Baez

Speech was still tough, but I was determined. I had to be strong and endure practicing long words even when they were not right at first. I was still working with blocks to say multisyllabic words better. The words that I worked on were dreary, thatch, vicinity, university, fluorescent, frequently, frustration, satisfy, punctual, historian, and physical. My speech session was intense and exhaustive. I felt stretched to the limit, but I kept plodding on.

Brain Attack

The effort to speak again wore me out.

A nurse friend gave me the following story:

About ten years ago, a young, successful executive named Josh was driving down a street and was going a bit too fast in his sleek, black, 12-cylinder Jaguar XKE, which was only two months old.

He watched for kids darting out from between parked cars and slowed down when he thought he saw something. As he passed a parked car, a brick sailed out and smashed into his car door! He slammed on the brakes, gears ground into reverse, and the Jaguar stopped where the brick had been thrown. Josh jumped out of the car, grabbed the kid who had thrown the brick, and shouted at him, "What was that all about. and who are you? Just what the heck are you doing?" Building up a head of steam, he went on, "That's my new Jaguar. That brick you threw is gonna cost you a lot of money. Why did you throw it?".

"I threw the brick because no one else would stop!" the boy said. Tears were dripping down the boy's chin as he pointed around the parked car. "My brother fell out of his wheelchair, and I can't lift him up. He's hurt, and he's too heavy for me."

It was a long walk back to his car, and Josh never did fix the door of his Jaguar. He keeps the dent to remind him not to go through life so fast that someone had to throw a brick at him to get his attention. Some bricks are softer than others.

I had been hit by a brick with this stroke. I guess it was part of my life lesson. I did know that my Number One priority was to speak well again privately and publicly.

Sue

Polly called me and asked if I could give her lecture in Chicago in June if she couldn't give it. I knew that I could never fill her shoes, and I couldn't believe that Polly was considering me as a replacement. On the phone, Polly's spirit and sense of humor were apparent and were still a part of her. I know the conversation was as hard for Polly as it was hard for me to be patient and allow her to finish her thoughts.

April 23, 1999

There is no such thing as a problem
without a gift for you in its hands.
A Course in Miracles

I awoke at 4 am and couldn't get back to sleep. I sat stewing about the speaking engagements that I needed to do for the year. I used to give five speeches in a day, but I didn't see how I would be able to keep that pace again. I knew that I would have to tell conference coordinators in Phoenix that I couldn't give the two-day seminar I had scheduled in the fall – more people who would have to be told that I was unable to do something. I had prided myself on the way that I could organize my speaking schedule. As I sat there, I had to remember that my life would never be the same.

So many people were depending on me. I had so much weight on my shoulders, that I felt as if I weighed a thousand pounds. Each lecture added more weight to my frame. I hoped my shoulders wouldn't break.

I had to get my life into manageable chunks. It didn't feel manageable yet. I understood why people describe a mental breakdown in those words. Life must have been too much for them. I just told myself that I could do anything, and this too would pass.

Lurking in the recesses of my brain was the issue of money. I was in a bind. I couldn't resolve money issues until I could work, but I couldn't work yet. What would I do until I could? Into my mind popped an image of a commercial in which a woman in a bubble bath says, "Calgon, take me away." I wanted someone to take this problem away from my consciousness. That is what I did by sleeping, but sleeping didn't always work. I couldn't do much more.

I started writing intensely to help get my feelings out. As I was writing and thinking, a new day dawned. Through my living room window where just a few minutes before there had been darkness, I could see the shadows of the mountains. The sky had many hues, from light blue to lavender to vivid blue. The colors had a hazy glow. Just a moment before, the trees were ill-defined shapes, and now they had come into focus. I could see definition in the branches. They had nubby bark, and they swayed in the wind.

As the wind blew the night away, I could see the core of my life. I had to refocus my life like a set of field glasses that had been askew.

I was tired of recovery, but I refused to cry, until I could decide what to do. I couldn't grieve over the splintered remnants of my past life until I knew what to do with the current one. In my mind I saw the image of a shattered Christmas ornament.

During the day, I called a magazine editor about an article I had written that was missing my byline. I didn't make any mistakes when I talked to the editor. That felt good. Now I have to keep doing it.

In the evening Eric came home with a bouquet of flowers for me. He said that they were for the hard work that I was doing with multisyllable words. A small gust of happiness floated through the room every time I glimpsed the bouquet. I was determined to build a new mosaic of words from the shards left after the stroke. The flowers validated my efforts and helped me work harder.

April 24, 1999

I hadn't eaten yet, and I was having trouble reading. I work so hard that I forget to eat in the morning.

Eric fixed the Lladro sculpture of a nurse holding a baby that I broke this week because I couldn't feel part of my hand. I am still very clumsy.

I walked two miles in 17 minutes. I'm getting faster. After walking on the treadmill I had to rest before I could do my homework for the day.

When I answered the phone, I had to repeat "Cutting Edge Press" in my mind so I could say it right. I left a voice-mail message for a customer in the morning. This was the first time I had correctly spoken all the words in the message, including numbers. Numbers had been an anathema to me. I had practiced saying the numbers in a phone number or zip code. Saying numbers quickly was so hard. Writing them quickly was also a problem, but I had to get better with that so I could take orders in our business.

I can read faster in the morning than at night, so I spent about an hour or so practicing multisyllable words again.

April 25, 1999

A woman is like a tea bag:
You never know her strength until you drop her in hot water.
Eleanor Roosevelt

I had a tug-of-war with words, when I said words for 35 or 45 minutes. Most people didn't know what an effort it took to talk. It seemed like I was pushing marbles out of my mouth one sound at a time. My jaw hurt from saying so many words. By the end of the session, the words were winning. Sometimes I'm envious of the things that most people take for granted, like speaking.

I had a huge list of words for Donna that I wanted to be able to say.

I was overtired most of the time. I guess my brain was using all my energy to relearn how to speak.

April 26, 1999

Teachers open the door, but you must enter by yourself.
Chinese Proverb

Sometimes I felt that I was pounding on the door of my overcrowded mind when I worked on the enormous number of words that I wanted to be able to say. They included:

tractor	reaction	properly	hydrangea	territory	thatch
dreary	university	vicinity	zoological	theft	vocabulary

April 27, 1999

More words that I wanted to say:

futility	representative	veterinarian	zealousness	zippiness
fluorescent	frequently	stretchable	stupendous	neurological
qualification	frustration	innocent	technique	auspicious
continuation	audiologist	historian	tendency	satisfy

April 28, 1999

One of the sweetest things in life: the letter of a friend.
Andy Rooney

One of my intuitive friends sent me an e-mail asking me how I was doing. She said that even though she hadn't talked with me on the phone, she felt that I was better overall and that the talking was clicking better too. She was right. How did she know that?

Chapter Nine
Spring Brings New Life

May 1, 1999

One day in the country is worth a month in town.
C. Rossetti

Spring brought new life to the picture here. I was getting much joy watching the bulbs I planted in the fall burst into bloom. Just being able to describe the scene was an amazing achievement to me now. In the first month after the stroke, I couldn't think what even to call this process of unfolding. I had lost my ability to describe everything.

In those early days, when Donna would ask me to describe an object, there was nothingness in my mind. Sometimes I could describe a particular thing, but more often I couldn't. She gave me clues until I could think of something. As I wrote this journal entry, I felt lucky to able to describe things more richly.

I decided that I would write the speech that I was to give in Chicago on empowerment. The writing went well, but it made me apprehensive because I knew that having written the speech, I had to try to give it. I had to face my fear of public speaking no matter how frightening it felt. I was reinventing myself.

May 2, 1999

Nothing in the world can take the place of perseverance.

Talent will not; nothing is more common than unsuccessful men with talent.

Genius will not; unrewarded genius is almost a proverb.

Education will not; the world is full of educated derelicts.

Persistence and determination are omnipotent.

Press on!

Calvin Coolidge

Brain Attack

The past two weeks were hard. I deleted some of my book, not once but twice, by pressing the wrong key on the computer. The mistake was partly a result of my poor motor planning. I felt as if I had lost my words again, because I needed a long time to start writing. But I decided that life isn't about what happens to you, but about how you deal with it, so I started writing again.

When I walked on my treadmill, I said the speech that I would give in Chicago. It was about an hour long. I was always good at focusing on a goal, and I would see if I could still do it with the speech.

May 3, 1999

Many of us spend our whole lives running from feeling
with the mistaken belief that you cannot bear the pain.
But you have already borne the pain.
What you have done is feel all you are beyond the pain.
Kahlil Gibran

In speech therapy, I asked Donna if I should do the AWHONN speech on empowerment. I felt so strongly about the topic, I felt called to do it. I figured that Donna would say it was too soon because I had the stroke only five months before. I had the surprise of my life when she replied that it wasn't too soon to try.

So I said the whole speech, and she said she thought I could do it. Oh dear, I had given myself a deadline, and that felt really intimidating. Now I had to get cracking to meet the deadline in June. Was this too ambitious a goal?

May 6, 1999

The greatest accomplishment is not in never falling,
but in rising after you fall.
Vince Lombardi

My speech session got off to a rough start. I think that was because I was doubting my ability to give the lecture. My gut and heart told me that the time was right, but my brain kept yelling, "Whoa!" I knew in my heart that giving the speech was the best thing to do. I just needed moral support.

Donna asked what I was afraid of. I was afraid of getting up in front of an audience and not being able to speak. I was afraid of having bitten off too much when I said that I would give the lecture. I was afraid of failing even though I always told my sons that if you don't try you know what you will get – nothing.

Rehabilitation is about reconditioning the body to inhabit the world in a different way. Until now, I was going through the motions of rehab. Now began the healing of my soul. I was working hard to "be in the moment" and to be aware of all my thoughts and actions. I seemed to do better when I stayed in the present. My priorities became clearer and clearer, but it was when I thought about the future that I began to worry.

I was practicing the speech on empowerment while I was walking on my treadmill. One word got jumbled up and came out "brank," the single word I could say after the stroke. Hearing myself say that word was like a bomb dropping out of the sky. It summoned up all the feelings I had experienced when I had the brain attack.

I wouldn't trade my life with anyone even though the stroke had complicated it. A lot of the time I was optimistic and positive, but there were some days when I wanted to pull the covers over my head, stay in bed, and pretend that this was all a bad dream.

My second son sent me a Mother's Day gift. He always takes his time at choosing gifts, and I cried when I opened it. It was a heart-shaped vase that he had made and painted himself. On the front he had written, "My mom is my hero." The accompanying card said, "I love you and am very proud of you." When he reads this, he'll know how much that meant to me. When I doubt myself, I look at the vase.

May 7, 1999

Music washes away from the soul the dust of everyday life.
Berthold Auerbach

I practiced my speech twice today and made a list of the hard words in it. I practiced them three times before I went to bed.

By 9:30 pm I was having a hard time reading. I had to concentrate hard just to read one sentence. I guess my body was telling me to go to bed.

I sent the speech to my friend Ana to read as I was worried about giving it. I have never been scared about giving a speech before. That was a new emotion for me.

I haven't enjoyed music for a long time. Right after the stroke, I couldn't stand to hear any kind of music because it made me feel anxious, and I would ask people to turn it off. The first time I realized that I would like to hear music again was a few weeks earlier when I went out to dinner with friends. I spent today by myself and put on a CD of the Dixie Chicks while I worked on my speech. I tried to enunciate my words clearly, loudly, and precisely.

I had been good at meeting deadlines, and this speech felt like a deadline. I was working like a Trojan horse on the project.

FROM THE SPEECH PATHOLOGIST

Polly attacked the task of giving a speech with the energy of a dynamo. She worked on writing, speaking, putting slides together with the text, voice, inflection, volume, prosody, rhythm, fluency – we practiced the speech daily. For the first time, Polly said to me, "I think I hear my old voice there once in a while...it is there." I had listened to tapes of several of Polly's speeches and I had read her books in an effort to capture the essence of her verbal and written style. She was a powerful and dynamic speaker. Even when I didn't know anything about the subject matter, it was obvious that she was captivating. She had a rapid, sure-fire delivery with incredible flexibility and ease. As she stated, she never read a speech; she worked only with notes or sometimes with nothing at all. Her ability to stay on track and deliver the message was awe-inspiring. We certainly had our work cut out for us.

I also knew that what Polly was doing was only a first step toward recovering her speaking ability. She had the courage and the will to get up and try. That was inspiring for all of us. While we didn't know Polly before the stroke, we knew that someone very special was now influencing our lives.

May 8, 1999

Risk everything, or gain nothing.
Geoffrey de Charney, 1358

I had a distressing dream about the worst imaginable errors a public speaker can make. I tried to not remember the dream because I didn't want it to come true. The dream was swimming in my brain, but I didn't want to confront the issues it raised.

I used imagery a lot after the stroke – trying to visualize what I wanted to do. You see yourself doing something correctly before you do it. It was something my gymnast son always did just before he started a meet. I formed a mental picture of words and tried to spell and pronounce them as I saw them in my mind. I also used imagery to help my recall.

I didn't feel so lost in my skin now. Before, it seemed to me that I didn't know where my body was in space.

I said the speech two times and the hard words about ten times. I took Donna's advice about exaggerating all my words and sounds. She also told me to speak loudly as it would help my fluency.

I had asked Eric to help me improve my flower beds, and this was a nice day for gardening. This was the first time since the stroke that I worked in my yard.

May 9, 1999

Hope is the thing with feathers

That perches on the soul

And sings the tune without the words

And never stops at all.

Emily Dickinson

Happy Mother's Day

I said the speech three times: for Eric in the house and on the phone for my mother and father and for one of my sons. I was still trying to learn to say the words clearly. I kept asking Eric if I could give the speech in a month, and his fervent belief was that I can do public speaking again.

When I wanted to remember something, I repeated the phrase in my mind.

Sometimes when I talked, it seemed that I was doing a monkey dance and just imitating others.

I tried not to take the brain attack so seriously. Occasionally I did something that was so funny that I had to laugh at myself even though it was sad. Saying my son's name and having it come out "Sex" was one of those things. I still laughed at that, but it also made me sad.

My speech-therapy sessions had a cozy, womb-like quality, as at last I felt safe there trying to speak. The amazing thing was that the more I opened up with Donna and was honest with her about my fears, the more my efforts to talk came together and the more progress I made.

May 10, 1999

Our first teacher is our own heart.
Cheyenne saying

I said the speech three times again. I was consumed with learning to say it.

I practiced all the words that were really difficult for me. I went through them about ten times while I was relaxing in the tub. When I got something in my head, I had to do it until it was right. But when I couldn't say the word "accomplishment," I had it, and I shouted "I hate this." I had shouted that sentence many times in the past five months. My anger was like bubbles that rise to the surface in boiling water. They pop open and then form again.

May 11, 1999

My doctors told me I would never walk again.
My mother told me I would.
I believed my mother.
Wilma Rudolph

I dreamed about public speaking again. In my dream, I could talk as I used to. Then I awoke and stammered and mispronounced words and couldn't think what I wanted to say.

Donna's office felt like a cocoon where I was safe and unjudged.

Bryan

I know that everyone was concerned when my mother announced that she was going to give her first public speech. What if she screws up? What if she freaks out? I thought it was a little early, but I knew that the milestone was important to her. I didn't say anything about its being too early. I knew that she was going to do it her way anyway. Typical!

May 13, 1999

We find in life exactly what we put into it.
Ralph Waldo Emerson

I had said the speech so many times that it made me sick, and it was not right yet. Before the stroke, I could have prepared the presentation in an afternoon. I had been laboring on this for days and still had more to do until I could be satisfied that it was my best.

One of my on-line friends told me that she was so excited that the woman her students quoted in their papers would be standing before her in a few weeks talking about empowerment. This note gave me the impetus to keep practicing the speech even though I was sick of it.

May 14, 1999

When you get in a tight place and everything goes against you,
till it seems as though you could not hold on a minute longer,
never give up then, for that is just the place
and time that the tide will turn.

Harriet Beecher Stowe

In the evening I gave an off-the-cuff speech about obstetrics at a doula training in Burlington organized by my friend Penny. It was a small group – 25 or 30 women. I wasn't nervous, and I kept wondering why not. But as long as I've been a public speaker, I've never been nervous. I asked myself what would be the worst thing that could happen to me during the talk. The answer was not being able to say anything. That seemed unlikely, so I just went ahead and gave the talk.

I held my own in a discussion with Penny, and then we fielded about two hours' worth of questions. Someone asked me how I felt, and I answered, "as if an old friend had come home." My occupational therapist Debbie drove me to Burlington because the meeting was at night. She said I was awesome.

Donna suggested that I decrease my speech therapy from five times a week to three. My fear was that I wouldn't get well faster with fewer sessions. Someways it felt as if I was being penalized for getting better.

"Is the decrease in sessions like the mama bird's telling the baby bird that he can fly?" I asked Donna. "Are you sure that I won't fall to the ground?" Donna said that the analogy about the bird was appropriate. She said that I did have wings, and she believed I could fly!

She told me that she couldn't promise that I wouldn't fall to the ground, but she would go with an 80 percent guarantee. She told me that once I was flying, I might have a few moments of feeling that I might fall down to tree level, but I would be safe in the branches if I faltered.

Brain Attack

May 15, 1999

Reach high, for the stars lie hidden in your soul.
Dream deep, for every dream precedes the goal.
Pamela Vaull Starr

In the morning I spoke again to the doula meeting about communicating with nurses and doctors – essentially my reflections on being both a nurse and a doula. I was told that it should last 20 to 25 minutes, but I was on a roll and I kept talking for about twice that time. I had trouble with a few words but, all in all, the applause told me the speech was received well. The clapping was good to hear. I taped the speech and listened to it later, and I felt good about it.

Many people said that I was an inspiration for them. I never know what to answer to that. People acted as if I had done something incredible, but I don't think I did. I had been frustrated sometimes during the past five months, but I created what I wanted. I was used to competing with myself; sometimes I was my fiercest competitor.

I told myself that I was going to get better faster than most people do. If I get something in my mind, I follow through. Eric says, "Don't get in Polly's way when she wants something."

Donna said that she knew that I wouldn't have a problem with the two sessions and that I was truly on my way. I was glad that she and my family and friends believed in me. One of my Houston friends wrote to me that it wasn't bad for a chick who had had a stroke less than six months ago.

Penny

I wrote to Polly in February and received a card from her that looked as if it were written by a five-year-old. I also talked with Polly a couple of times and was impressed with how well she did, even though she groped for words at times and her speech was hesitant.

In April I invited her to speak at a doula training I was doing in Burlington in May. I knew she was working hard to regain her speaking ability, and I thought a half hour talk might be a way to "break in" again on the speaking circuit (as well as inspire the future doulas).

Her talk in May was very well received; it included lessons to be learned from her stroke experience and material on the relationship between nurses and doulas. Polly's sense of humor continued throughout the time she spent with me. Her story touched and inspired everyone in the doula world.

May 16, 1999

A ship in the harbor is safe, but that's not what ships are for.

My right foot is only something that holds me up. I long for the time when I can feel my toes rubbing each other.

May 18, 1999

You'll learn more about a road by traveling it than by looking at maps.

In answer to my letter to her about the talk, a friend of mine wrote, "Keep up the good work. You are not only getting back to normal, you are getting better." When I read it, I realized that she was right. This episode in my life made me take stock of what was really important to me and cracked open my inner world for me to examine. My struggles had already given much to me, particularly the friendships I made because of the brain attack.

I got frustrated today about some of the plans for my trip to Chicago. I couldn't get a room in the convention hotel, and the only help the organizers gave me was the suggestion that I stay in a hotel far from the convention and take a cab. When I told the organizers that those arrangements would be difficult for me, they essentially shrugged and said, "We hope you'll be able to give the speech." I was at last able to arrange to share a room with a colleague. I had been working so hard on the speech for the convention that this glitch, which once would have seemed so minor, felt enormous to me. I screamed out loud. I could not keep my emotions inside.

May 19, 1999

To the question of your life, you are the only answer.
To the problem of your life, you are the only solution.
Jo Coudert

I was trying to give myself time to get used to the realities of life after a stroke, as I considered what I had to change in order to work again. The answer was a lot. Every time I made a plan or a commitment, I had to take the stroke into account.

Brain Attack

In a phone call, someone I'm close to told me I was trying to do too much. When I explained that I had to work hard to speak again, the retort was, "If you want to have another stroke, go ahead." The comment upset me so much that I needed to talk to one of my friends about it. She wasn't home, so I left her a voice message. When she called me back, she said, "Do you realize that when you left your message, you didn't say any words incorrectly even though you were crying?"

May 20, 1999

God, I've been starving for this kind of conversation!
Eleanor Coppola

I spent the evening with two of my friends and felt for the first time since the stroke that I was a part of the conversation. My friends always tried to include me, but I didn't feel that I could talk well enough to participate, and I only listened when they talked.

May 21, 1999

The way I see it, if you want the rainbow,
you gotta put up with the rain.
Dolly Parton

Driving to Jane's in the morning, I practiced one of the sentences from my Chicago speech: "Life is not inherently safe." I said it right several times. That one sentence had been giving me a hard time, and I felt good to be able to say it right.

All day I felt that I was saying multisyllable words better. I should have felt better, but in some ways I felt worse because I feared my progress wouldn't continue. I wanted to fill the spaces between words with melodious sound, but the gaps in my speech remained.

I practiced the words that Donna gave me including: strup, strap, strep, strop, plump, prep, plop, plow, smell, snare, snow, clip, clap, clop, and clup. The exercise made me think back to several months before, when the ground was covered with snow and I couldn't say the word "snow" no matter how much I wanted to.

May 22, 1999

When I had dinner with friends and everyone was talking, I felt as if I wasn't there. I felt a strong reaction to some people's words, and it may not have had anything to do with the situation at hand. I was trying to stop, wait, and get clear about what this was all about. Perhaps it was part of a letting go process. My life will never be the same, but I wish I could figure out what it will be.

Tired as I was, if I wanted to work again, I had to endure the re-learning process. Nighttime was when I lost my control, usually because I was tired.

May 23, 1999

At the core of life is hard purposefulness,
a determination to live.
Howard Thurman

The process of writing was still terribly hard. I had to search for the word I wanted to write and then say it aloud to myself. Spelling a word right took a long time. Trying to spell the word "scrap," for example, elicited strap, scap, and scarp before I got the spelling right. If I thought I had spelled a word wrong, I enlisted Eric's help if he was home. If he wasn't, I used spell check on the computer. Sometimes this didn't work either, and then I tried to find the right spelling on a hand-held spelling device that Donna lent me called Spelling Ace. If this all didn't work, I had to either scrap the word or sentence or try to write it in a different way.

Among the things I was trying to write were e-mail comments to colleagues on a perinatal list-serve. After the stroke, I read others' comments, but I usually said nothing in reply. I was giving my comments again on various topics – many related to seeing medicine through the eyes of the patient and not of the nurse.

Sue

Polly's comments to the perinatal nurse internet list were incredible and reminded us about the role nurses play in our patients' lives. Her tone had changed from research to real-life experience. I was devastated by the cruelties she endured in the hospital from professionals who were supposed to be nurturing and caring. As a nurse, I have long been angry with so-called good nurses, who were technically competent but didn't support patients' emotional needs. Polly's experience could happen to any of us.

Brain Attack

May 24, 1999

You cannot discover new oceans
unless you have the courage to lose sight of the shore.
C. Cheng

My self-confidence began to wane, for no reason that I could pinpoint. It just happened. Some days I feel that I can do anything, and other days I feel like an idiot. The bad days are worse when I'm tired or frustrated. I needed guidance and direction. I hated sounding like a monotone fool, so I liked working on inflection in speech therapy.

I was tired of people finishing my sentences. If I was going to speak better, I needed to try to say words. I know that people want to help me, but when they jumped in and said the words they thought I was trying to say, they were sometimes right and other times pitifully wrong. I usually didn't care at that point, and I just quit and felt lost. If people want to help me, they need to help me try to say things myself..

In rehab on Thursday, I'll give the speech I've prepared for Chicago. I feel like I'm going to work again. Eric, Jane, and Michael will be out of town. I'll celebrate without them.

May 25, 1999

You've got to have a dream,
if you don't have a dream,
how you gonna have a dream come true?
Oscar Hammerstein

Looking for a word that I want to say is like dancing with a shadow. I envy those who can speak with abandon. I wonder if my speech will be forever dull and flat.

I received many remarkable notes and cards from people I didn't even know but who had heard about me from colleagues on the Internet. Their generosity with their time overwhelmed me.

May 27, 1999

Success is not measured by what a man accomplishes,
but by the opposition he has encountered,
and the courage with which he maintained
the struggle against overwhelming odds.

Charles A. Lindbergh

Today I gave my AWHONN speech for some of the people who work in rehab at the hospital. Again I was surprised that I wasn't nervous. I made some last-minute preparations as I have always done before giving a speech. The whole outpatient department came to hear me.

When I started speaking, I felt amazingly calm. I had to measure my words carefully, and in some ways that made my words stronger. There were fewer words, but they were powerful.

Getting a compliment from your speech therapist about the first speech that you give after a stroke is a great feeling, a feeling that carried me for a long time.

One of my friends took me out for supper to celebrate. It was a wonderful end of the day good food, good wine, a good friend, and a toast to the future.

FROM THE SPEECH PATHOLOGIST

Polly was ready to speak in public again. She delivered an inspirational message to the Rehab Department. The staff was flabbergasted at her improvement. She was on her way.

Marje

I watched Polly work so hard on her speech, saying it over and over until she felt it was right. Listening to her today, we were moved, not so much by what she said but by how passionately she said it. Her words came from her heart, and that was immediately felt by everyone in the room. It was truly a lesson in recovery.

May 28, 1999

Sometimes before I tried to talk, there was a calm before the storm. Multiple sounds danced in my head. As I got better, the sounds danced tighter together, and they converged into a word.

FROM THE SPEECH PATHOLOGIST

Polly was on her way, but we still had a long way to go. Polly's fluency had improved, but apraxia had a way of sneaking in, especially when Polly was tired or hadn't eaten.

May 30, 1999

The times are a-changing.
Bob Dylan

It was beautiful outside this weekend. When I got up in the morning, I sat on the deck right outside of my bedroom and read. Fabulous!

Then I exercised on the treadmill while saying the AWHONN speech for the umpteenth time. I had made some additions and had to learn to say the new words correctly. I tried to feel my tongue when it cradled the words like a pillow cradles the head. The speaking stuff was still very complicated to me. I wanted so badly to say words that I could have pulled my hair out.

I could feel my right ear for the first time since the stroke. It itched and felt weird and prickly.

Chapter Ten
First Professional Speech

June 1, 1999

The tune and refrain of the Beatles song, "It's getting better all the time," reverberates in my mind. Maybe because I am getting better.

I suddenly realized how vulnerable I will be if I make my innermost thoughts public in a book. I will be exposed, and this is very forbidding because I am usually very private with strangers. In my work I am outgoing, but that writing is factual not personal. Sometimes I want to keep my journal personal, but it might help someone else. This is an inner struggle for me.

June 2, 1999

Give sorrow words.
William Shakespeare

The trees I see through my window are in full leaf. It has been six months since my brain attack and the start of my new life.

I cherish tranquil moments, but they are scarce. It seems as if I have been working every second since I had the stroke, and I'm so tired. I wish that things would slow down, but I've got so much to do to be able to speak fluently.

I spent 30 minutes talking with the accounting department at the hospital about my bill. That was a feat in itself. At first the woman talked to me as if I was an idiot. When I told her that I had worked in the health-care field for 35 years, her manner changed. I reminded her that I had been unemployed for the last six months because of the stroke. I didn't have a clue as to how I could get the money to pay so huge a bill. A conversation ensued about the charges. She told me to talk with my therapists. I gently reminded her that they didn't have anything to do with the charges, but the business office did.

The whole conversation was physically and emotionally difficult, and I knew that it was far from over. The conversation caused me a crisis in confidence because I was treated like a poor stroke victim even though I knew what I was talking about, maybe even more than the person I was talking to.

I had trouble controlling the volume of my voice. Since it was harder to speak loudly than to speak softly, I often spoke in a monotone. I hope that

135

with time, I'll learn inflection again. I speak more softly than before the stroke, because I think that I might make a mistake. I have learned more about articulation than I wanted to know.

Donna told me that the latest version of the empowerment speech with slides was good. In my rational brain, I knew she was right. Donna talked about the things I had to do to get ready to give the speech. They had more to do with delivery, such as inflection and tone, than about content. I was not fishing for compliments when I said to Donna, "I guess that this is not too bad for six months after a stroke." Her reply was, "I'd say it is more than good – it's amazing." Being able to give the speech gave me a sense of achievement, even if it might contain some mispronounced words.

I tried to say my speech two times at night, but I kept making mistakes. I railed on about my inability to speak the words in my presentation clearly. I dissolved into tears for the millionth time. I threw up my hands, shouting, "I hate this! I hate this!" I didn't want to whine, but that's what I was doing. My fit wasn't over as I told my very patient husband, "You couldn't do this." He quietly replied, "This is very hard for you, but you will get better." I was glad to get that out. Most people don't have a clue how difficult this is.

I'm tired of exploring my emotional landscape. Will I ever be happy-go-lucky again?

June 3, 1999

Deal with the faults of others as gently as with your own.
Chinese Proverb

I can feel the palm of my hand now, but my fingers can't feel one another's sides. Sometimes I can grip a bottle I need to open, and then sometimes I can't.

Today I gave the Chicago speech for Donna again, and I felt so tired because the amount of energy I need in order to speak is enormous. My mouth hurts as it does after a trip to the dentist. When I try to speak, it seems that there are too many words for me to choose from, and none of them are right. In my mind, doors appear. The problem is knowing which door has the right word.

I have to get used to speaking slowly. And I used to speak for a full day all the time.

I still have trouble saying numbers and finding the page in a magazine where an article continues. It is still hard to look up anything alphabetically.

June 4, 1999

There are risks and costs to a program of action.
But they are far less than the long range risks
and costs of comfortable inactions.
John Fitzgerald Kennedy

For the first time since the stroke, I felt water hitting my right foot in the shower in the morning. Until then, I could feel that something was on my foot, but I couldn't tell what it was. Now I can tell when beads of water are cascading down my foot.

Sometimes when I need to say words, I feel like a magician with a bunny in a hat. Coming up with the right word is like pulling out the rabbit. After I say the word, I want to say, "ta-da," and actually I do say it sometimes because finding the word feels so monumental to me.

June 5, 1999

Take care of the present, and the future will take care of itself.
Ross Greene, PhD

I still have good days and bad days. I wish I could read better at night. I still can't do things that require a lot of concentration. One of the reasons that I get up early is that I know I'm at my best after a good night's sleep. I used to be a night-owl. I wonder if I'll feel carefree ever again.

June 8, 1999

The best thing about the future is that it only
comes one day at a time.
Abraham Lincoln

Donna discussed her goals for me. There were a lot of them. I have to work on:
- strategies for using numbers
- exercises for complex and abstract words
- rate of speech and prosody of spontaneous speech
- using compensatory strategies during five-minute spontaneous conversation
- varying pitch in speech
- increasing fluency when reading aloud
- writing numbers from dictation
- self-monitoring in spontaneous conversation

They make me think I'll take forever to accomplish them. Sometimes I wish I didn't have to work so hard all the time. I asked Eric, "What do you think I'll be like in a year?" He said, "You'll be perfect!"

June 9, 1999

Brains first and then hard work.
Eeyore – Pooh's Little Instructional Book

My right ankle and foot finally feel like part of my body. My foot used to feel like a phantom limb. I could walk, but something was missing and I didn't know what.

Usually you have time to savor the moment, but I'm afraid that if I do that I will lose time. I feel that I'm running out of time – not time to work on the speech, which is in four days, but time to get better. I know that our insurance won't last much longer, and then I won't have the help I need to speak better.

I want to take a vacation from this rehab, but I know I can't. I keep telling myself not to be so hard on myself, but I'm afraid of not having enough time. It may not be rational, but I still feel this way.

June 12, 1999

All that we see or seem
is but a dream within a dream.
Edgar allen Poe

Two days before my first speech before a large audience since the stroke, I was psychologically exhausted. I had been on a roller coaster of emotions for the past three days. Most people can't understand how difficult it is to do something over and over until you hate it so much you want to scream, but you have to keep doing it. That was why I kept practicing the speech. The impression I give the nurses is so important. I want them to see that we who have suffered a stroke can get well and do the work we love. I also want them to see that I can still give my listeners their money's worth. My speaking reputation hangs on this speech. With so much going on, I felt anxious and apprehensive. I got up really early and walked on the treadmill to calm the stress demons.

Then my flight to Chicago was canceled. I'll get there tomorrow. Strangely enough, I didn't mind the cancellation. I liked having the extra day. I was tired of practicing the speech, and I filled the day with mindless activity – cleaning my office.

June 13, 1999

Do not fear risk.

All exploration is calculated.

Only if we are willing to walk over the edge can we become winners.
The families of the Challenger Shuttle Crew, –
One year after the disaster.

After working so brutally hard preparing the speech for AWHONN, I tried to stay relaxed and focused on the trip. I slept well, but I got up early to give myself time to get ready without hurrying. I did give Eric a hard time leaving for the airport early – he's almost always close to missing a plane.

Eric drove me to the airport in Burlington where I found that my seat was changed because of the change in schedule. The airline agent was trying to explain the changes to me, but he talked too fast. That frustrated me because I need a lot of time to process what someone is saying. He treated me as if I was dumb, but in my usual fashion I told him, "I have had a stroke, and it takes me longer to understand what you are saying, but I am not dumb." He became nicer then. I have no trouble telling people I had a stroke.

The trip through O'Hare airport went fine, and I found the shuttle to the hotel easily. I listened to another speaker in the afternoon. Will I ever be able to speak as easily as she did?

I went to hear a friend give the keynote address, but I couldn't find a vacant chair, and I sat on the floor. When the speaker began, she projected a slide on the screen, but I couldn't see it from where I was sitting. Then I heard my name, and I stood up to see the slide. It was a picture of me. She said how hard I had been working to give my speech. It was such a sweet thing to do. I was flabbergasted.

Time was winding down. My expectations and the last sixth months of speech therapy were on the line. No time for self-doubt, but I was faced with the tension between roots and wings: Part of me wanted to stay rooted safely on the ground, but another part of me wanted to soar.

I checked out the room where I was going to speak. Then I practiced the speech again.

Brain Attack

June 14, 1999

Life isn't a matter of milestones. But of moments.

Rose Kennedy

I woke up early. The morning was fraught with tension as I practiced the hardest parts of the speech again. To give myself a break, I went down to breakfast. I knew I had to eat well in order to speak well. In the restaurant I ran into the friend who had mentioned me in her speech the night before. It was serendipitous that she was there, because I needed to relax and chatting with her over breakfast relaxed me. Then I went back to my room and practiced the hardest words in the speech.

I knew that I wasn't as good a speaker as I once was. I wanted to be as good a speaker as I could be at that moment. The information was in my brain; I hoped I would be able to get the right word to come out of my mouth.

I went to the lecture room early to check my slides. I worried that no one would come. At last, some people began coming in, and I spoke to some of them. I noticed my friend Roger standing at the back of the room. He has aphasia from a massive stroke and can say only a few words. Seeing him there made me more determined to make the speech good.

Then I went to the front of the room and sat down. A few colleagues and friends came up and talked to me. That helped me feel calm.

I decided that I would use some of the time allotted to introductions to teach about strokes. I had a captive audience, and I wanted to take advantage of it. Information about strokes could one day be important to the people in my audience or to their loved ones. So I asked the nurse who was to introduce me to tell a bit about strokes instead of rattling on about where I went to school. She agreed because Roger is her husband and because we are both nurses and educators with similar passions. She told about the many deficits I had after the stroke. As she spoke, I turned to a friend sitting beside me and joked that it was quite a long list.

Then it was show time.

I walked to the podium. There were 120 people filling the room to capacity, and one gutsy woman in front of them. I had a fierce energy inside me to make the speech good for the nurses in the audience and for myself. The topic of empowerment was so timely for me and for them. They were struggling with changes in health care, as I was struggling with trying to speak again.

I pulled the words of the speech right out of my heart. I said that I had had a large lesson in empowerment during the past year. I used slides that showed quotes that I used while I tried to learn to speak again. I wove the story of my stroke into the speech so that the nurses could see how important they could be to their patients. I talked about the nurses who took care of me and how they empowered me to recover after the stroke.

I said that as health-care professionals we had to take a risk. Life is not inherently safe. I took a risk in trying to save myself after the stroke. I took a risk trying to speak again. I took risks coming to Chicago to talk. I took a risk learning to write, spell, and do math again.

I told them that I have to think about every word I say. I take a risk every time I speak. But risk is in the eyes of the beholder. Our sense of risk is based on our fears.

When we say things are risky, we mean we are scared. Most of us are running away from what we are afraid of. Wouldn't it be better to run toward what we want?

Our fear contributes to the outcome of the risk and therefore to the risk itself. I asked the audience a question: Risk what? I implored them to risk being advocates. I told them that they must risk trying new ways of empowering themselves and others. They must help to create health not just treat disease, and they must empower their patients to do the same.

I asked the nurses to use all their skills – critical thinking, clinical judgement, assessment, and advocacy – to look at health care through their patients' eyes. How do patients feel? What do they need? Did a particular policy benefit the patient, or was it just a ritual?

I asked them to remember that they are the backbone of the medical system and to recognize how important they are to their patients. I urged them to build up one another, as we must enhance each others' unique qualities. I encouraged them to make flexibility a key concept in their practice. I asked them to dare to be different.

I closed by asking the nurses to dedicate themselves to including empowerment in their care and to listening to their inner voice. I told them that to follow the path to empowerment is to take a risk. But I had taken a risk, and I knew they could take a risk too.

I repeated the question: Risk what? And I told them that the answer was in each of them.

In the middle of the speech, I realized that everything was flowing for the gal who was not good at flowing. Against all odds I was giving my first speech after the brain attack. The moment was my triumph over adversity.

I stumbled over only a few words. I had wondered if I had it in me to give the talk. After I finished, I thought I had been marvelous. But what about the audience? Since I was so focused on saying the words correctly and with the right inflection, it took me a little time to hear the audience clapping. I was amazed when everyone stood up and applauded. The standing ovation was the fruit of my labor for the past six months.

As they say in Texas, "Yeee haaa!"

A few people came up to me after the speech. A nurse told me that her biggest fear was that she would have a stroke. After listening to me, she wasn't so afraid. Roger's wife brought tears to my eyes when she told me that during my speech Roger was nodding in agreement.

My trip home was difficult. When I got to O'Hare, I had trouble thinking amid the airport hustle and bustle. Crowds of people stood in many lines that snaked around the foyer. The airport was confusing before I had the stroke; after the brain attack, it was impossible. There were too many choices. Where was I supposed to go? What line should I get in? I finally decided to go to the gate to avoid the possibility of getting into the wrong line. At last I got to the right gate.

Celeste

I had the pleasure and honor of introducing Polly at the national AWHONN meeting. Her presentation before a large audience was inspiring, to say the least. After Polly's speech, one participant said to me, "This experience made coming to the convention worthwhile. The whole convention revolves around this one presentation. What an inspiration!"

Eric

Polly called me after she finished her speech in Chicago. She was surprised at the standing ovation, but I was not. I knew that people were just waiting to hear what she had to say and that they wouldn't care if she mispronounced a few words.

June 15, 1999

Courage is not the absence of fear,
but rather the judgement that something
else is more important than fear.

Ambrose Redmoon

I listened to a tape of yesterday's speech. It had a few bobbles, but I thought it was good for my first effort in public speaking since the stroke. I reflected that for me speaking is always a concious and deliberate act. It is not automatic, and most times it is exhausting.

I was relieved to have the first major speech under my belt. The audience made me feel that everything would turn out splendidly, and the standing ovation was a thrill. I felt that everyone there was proud of me, my courage, and my effort for the past six months. Now it's back to rehab and more challenges.

My right thigh had been aching for a week. I guess it was the nerves regenerating. I got myself a massage as a present for giving the speech well.

At night I was so tired, I was whining. I guess I earned the right to whine if I wanted to.

MEDICAL NOTES

Massage has been used since the fifth century BC to relieve tension and encourage healing by promoting the flow of blood and lymph. Nerves are stimulated and muscles are stretched and loosened to keep them elastic.

MEDICAL NOTES

Central poststroke pain is likely caused by central nervous system changes from the cerebrovascular accident (CVA) and is almost always on the side affected by the CVA. The pain is usually described as numbness, tingling, aching, throbbing, pinching or tearing pain.

"Stroke Rehabilitation
Hayn, Margaret, and Tina Fisher–
Nursing 97, March 1997 "

FROM THE MASSAGE THERAPIST

I don't think I will ever forget when Polly entered my office. I expected a weak, somewhat helpless woman who had suffered a stroke . What I saw was anything but that. My first impression was of a woman who exhibited great determination mixed with pride, hurt, frustration, and deep sadness who didn't have time for the stroke. She was very precise in sounding out her words, all the while keeping her back straight and her head up high.

When I asked her if she had told her doctor that she was getting a massage, she answered that she hadn't thought of that because it wasn't his business. This scared me. My confidence was fading, and I wondered if she would work well with me.

Before the massage began, I told Polly about my plans to do light work. She wasn't happy with my decision. I think I added to her frustration. She wanted a massage that felt good and deep.

Luckily, I had called my massage instructor prior to Polly's visit to get advice about giving a massage to a person taking Coumadin. She assured me that if I did light work, the client would be fine.

My goal for the first session was to prevent joint stiffness along with relieving the constant muscle pain and stiffness associated with a stroke.

I wanted to ensure that the muscles surrounding the spine and extremities were loose and flexible, but it was important to achieve those results without bruising or rupturing blood vessels and producing blood clots. I called Polly after the session, and she reported that she was fine and the massage was helpful.

Jamie

Polly sent me the empowerment speech that she gave in Chicago, and I loved when she wrote, "It's not bad for a chick who couldn't talk six months ago." Her "voice" really came through.

June 16, 1999

***Painful as it may be, a significant emotional event can be the catalyst of choosing a direction that serves us – and those around us-more effectively.
Look for the learning.***

Eric Allenbaugh

It took me two days to rest from the speech. I felt like a limp rag. I had used every ounce of energy to speak fluently in Chicago. I took naps each day, even though napping is unusual for me. I was so relieved the speech was over.

I cried during my speech therapy session because I was doing what seemed to be a very hard exercise. When Donna asked why I was crying, I blubbered about being not able to take a break. I had worked every minute of the last months to regain my speech. Usually after you have done something hard, you get to savor it for awhile. I ended my crying and whining session by telling Donna I was so grateful that I could speak at all. Some stroke victims never can. I felt a mantle over my shoulders to speak the words that others couldn't. This was part of the lesson of the brain attack.

June 17, 1999

Difficulties are meant to rouse, not discourage.
William Ellery Channing

I am still navigating the tricky and challenging waters of the spoken word. Having apraxia is like living on a fault line. I never know if the ground might collapse beneath me when I have to say a word. I was heartened to receive an e-mail from a nurse who attended my session in Chicago. She told me that I was very eloquent for someone who couldn't speak six months earlier. I will hold her message in my heart for when the going gets tough.

June 19, 1999

Don't be afraid to take a big step when one is indicated.
You can't cross a chasm in two small jumps.
David Lloyd George

I've never been satisfied with the status quo. I decided this weekend to pronounce every one of the 300 words and phrases in the card set for apraxia therapy that Donna lent me. I had been working with the set since I was in the hospital. I bite down on a word and roll it around in my mouth until I can say it correctly. When I get a multi-syllable word right, I say it several times to savor it. I have always competed with myself. This is the only way I work. I had repeated all of the words and phrases individually, but today I challenged myself to say all of them.

Some days I feel that I'm getting the hang of this speaking thing, but on other days I wonder, "What am I doing?" I guess that this is one step back and two steps forward.

June 21, 1999

Every path serves a purpose.
Gene Oliver

I still watch Eric or Donna when they speak to see how their mouths work. With extra-difficult, polysyllabic words I ask them to repeat the words several times, and I watch as they say the words slowly and deliberately. I had to see and hear the words, especially if I hadn't said them before

My drive to speak again weighs heavily on me. I work hard to maintain the discipline I need to succeed. I did another set of 100 word cards as I was walking on the treadmill in the morning. I never ease up. My stamina amazes me sometimes. I don't know where this fortitude is coming from. It must have been deep in my soul. I've learned that I can be strong when I think there is no strength left inside of me.

I have become interested in the little things in life now. I like to watch the hummingbirds hover close to the flowers on my deck as their wings beat furiously.

FROM THE SPEECH PATHOLOGIST

Polly's spontaneous conversation was improving, but word retrieval was still a major issue. When Polly didn't have the words she wanted, she was often silent, and that was not good. This was an important juncture. Stroke patients who have difficulty with word retrieval are often reluctant to participate in conversations or to socialize for fear that they will have nothing to say or will say the wrong word.

June 22, 1999

One can present people with opportunities.
One cannot make them equal to them.
Rosamond Lehmann

One of my former monitrice clients in Houston called, and we chatted for about 30 minutes. She had thought that Eric would answer the phone, and she was surprised to hear me on the other end of the line. She said, "You sound fine to me." That was nice to hear because I thought that my conversational speech was better too. I worked late and my stamina seemed improved as well.

I told Donna that I felt as if I was working like a wild woman. When she laughed and I asked why, she retorted, "I've never seen you any other way."

Donna asked if I would talk to another woman who had a stroke. Of course I said, "Sure." I hope that assisting others will speed my own healing.

I was so busy that I only ate a peach and a plum until dinner. Then when some friends were here, I couldn't talk at all. That's what I got for not eating right.

June 24, 1999

I found out that my hospital bill had been turned over to a collection agency. I called the hospital and talked to a woman about my problems with my bill. She was the first person who seemed to care about my difficulties, and she told me to come to her office in the hospital so she could help me straighten out the billing mess. I told her that because I was self-employed, I couldn't pay until I could work again. I told her that giving my bill to a collection agency seemed like a bad move on their part. They are giving part of their money away. Until I can work again, there's no way for me to pay that huge bill. You can't get blood out of a turnip.

Donna asked me how I would feel about helping her start a stroke group in the area. I told her that I would help, if I didn't have to be the leader. I have spearheaded self-help groups before, but I didn't have the energy to take this on except as one of the followers. Although people tell me, "You're a good spokesperson for brain attacks," I don't want to be the poster girl for strokes. More and more, however, I am pulled in that direction. Right now I'm resisting, but then I feel that I need to help others. What a dilemma!

I told the Florida group that I would give a keynote address in October about comfort measures for women in labor. Even though I turned them down in April, the conference coordinator kept calling me. Whenever I expressed my fears, she would come up with a solution until I had no more excuses.

June 26, 1999

Life isn't about what happens to you,
but how you deal with what happens to you.
Benjamin-Bohm

I got a letter from the Social Security Administration denying my disability claim. It said that I wouldn't be disabled for a full 12 months and so wasn't entitled to any monetary compensation and that I should be able to do a menial task job that wouldn't involve the general public. I couldn't have even done that. I couldn't work in a restaurant because numbers were a black hole to me. I couldn't work on an assembly line because I was still easily confused. What did these people really know or care about me?

I never thought that I would get money from Social Security, but the wording in the letter depressed me. What happened to being optimistic and encouraging? Even though I thought that their pronouncement that I couldn't work with the general public was wrong, it still hurt my soul. I have worked every second since the stroke to regain my lost functions, and this edict told me to stop trying to work as a speaker. They stole my dream and my goal. It felt like a punch in the stomach, when I needed encouragement so badly. I was unprepared for the intensity of the feelings the letter aroused.

This week threw me a one-two punch with the letter and the lack of financial assistance from the hospital. I don't know if I can remain up-beat.

I need to start working on the Florida speech about comfort measures, but the letter made it more challenging because it told me not to set a goal like that. The letter left my ego so bruised and fragile. I was trying to shake the feeling of gloom it caused.

I needed guidance from God and from my own inner strength. So I repeated my mantra, "I can do anything!" Usually, hard work relieves my sense of frustration. I guess I just have to start working again.

June 27, 1999

I know God won't give me anything I can't handle.
But I just wish he didn't trust me so much.

Mother Teresa

Being patient is still not easy for me, so I hung up the "PATIENCE" paper that Marje made for my room in the hospital in Burlington. To remind me how far I have come since then, I looked at the homework I did right after the brain attack.

June 28, 1999

I saw Steve at the hospital, and he complimented me on my speaking. He jokes with me about my southern accent returning. If he can hear an accent, some of my inflection must be coming back. Donna noticed it too. In my speech session, when I said the word "git," she said, "I guess that's Texan for get, right?"

June 30, 1999

The reward of a thing well done is to have done it.
Ralph Waldo Emerson

There is an intensity in this experience that is hard to replicate. This life journey is like crossing a river by boat. At first my load was very heavy, and my friends and family lightened it by taking some of the pressures off me. Still I had too much weight in the boat, so my therapists helped by lightening the boat even more. Now if I want to get to the other side of the river, it's up to me to row the boat with the oars that I have.

Chapter Eleven
Facing Adversity

July 3, 1999

My parents sent me the nicest present: several gift certificates for massages to help ease the pain in my right leg. Without their gift, I wouldn't be able to get the massages that help me so.

I find that words are still mixed up in my mind, and often I can't think of the meaning of words that are in my head. When that happens I feel like I'm losing ground in my attempt to talk. I feel that if I can't say the words I want and don't know the meaning of other words, I can't go on, but in the next minute I shrug my shoulders and know that I must go on.

July 4, 1999

Music washes away from the soul the dust of everyday life.
Red Auerbach

I found myself singing along with the stereo this morning. It was a song called "Sister" from a vintage women's music album called "The Changer and the Changed" by Cris Williamson. That was the first time since the stroke that I could sing a song. I was so surprised that I started to cry.

My mom and dad called in the morning, and my mom said that they had listened to a tape of an incredible speaker. Eventually I realized that they were talking about my speech in Chicago. They said they were so proud of me. It made me smile.

July 6, 1999

My speech homework was to take four numbers, look at them for one to two seconds to memorize them, and then say them out loud. I had no trouble memorizing the numbers, but saying them was hard. For some reason, I had trouble visualizing numbers when I said them. If I said the word "table," I could picture a table, but numbers were too abstract. I wished that the numbers would glide off my tongue, but numbers were still hard for me to repeat quickly.

July 8, 1999

The day started on a bad note when I couldn't access one of the hard drives on my computer. I felt a sense of panic, which launched a multitude of tears. I wept inconsolably for half an hour. The problem with the hard drive recalled the time I erased part of this book in a computer error—not once but twice. Those mistakes made me feel as if I had dropped into a deep hole in the ground. Even now it is hard for me to write about the episode because after having lost my words in the stroke, I lost them twice again in the computer. When the hard drive failed, I felt the same sense of loss. It was like rewinding the tape in my brain and finding nothing on it.

I focused my fury on Eric and our mounting bills. I hadn't been crying over just a mistaken stroke on the keypad. The morning's tears were a symbol of my grief and pain over all that I had lost in the past seven months: my home in Houston, my Texas friends, the security of Eric's job, and everything the stroke had stripped from me—spelling, doing math, telling time, speaking without thinking.

July 9, 1999

In the face of adversity, never ever blink and never look back.

In one day, my mood changed dramatically for no reason other than the lability of my emotions. This was a day when I felt everything would be okay. I found an ad for Lee blue jeans that mirrored my philosophy. It said, "In the face of adversity, never ever blink and never look back." My new life is blossoming, as I am speaking better, especially multisyllable words. I am confident I will be able to do the work I love—motivating and empowering nurses. I won't let the stroke take that away from me. It doesn't matter how long it takes. Attitude is a powerful force.

FROM THE SPEECH PATHOLOGIST

I again called upon Polly to speak to a client who had been aphasic for several years. Polly rose to the challenge and was of considerable help just by telling my client how she felt about being aphasic and that she understood my client's struggle. All too often we think of the effects of a stroke in terms of physical, not verbal, paralysis, although verbal paralysis is often more debilitating and is frequently misunderstood by others. I have had so many language-disabled clients who were treated as if they were stupid because they couldn't respond or speak in sentences or with good grammar. With her typical strong sense of self, Polly told my client, "If they think I'm stupid because my grammar is not always right or I can't find a word, then that is their problem!"

July 10, 1999

I am trying to outsmart this illness called apraxia. I so want to have fluent speech that as I walked on my treadmill in the morning I said the 20 words on each of 50 apraxia cards. I was reminded of a poster that said, "The race belongs not only to the swift and strong but also to those who keep running." What if I am running on the wrong road?

When I can't pronounce a word that I want to say, a spasm of rage overtakes me. Sometimes I don't feel that I fit in anywhere.

July 11,1999

I said more words today while I exercised for an hour. I get so tired of the relentless, repetitive practice I need to do to be able to talk fluently, but I feel a passion for opening the door to the words in my mind.

My parents came for a visit and while they were here they met Donna. They wanted to thank her for working with me, and I wanted them to hear from her that I'm a hard worker and she was amazed at my progress.

Sometimes the families of stroke patients are concerned that any kind of exertion on the patient's part will cause another stroke. But stroke victims need to have as normal a life as possible under the circumstances, and coddling them only interferes with their independence. A neurologist can advise whether the family's concern is warranted.

July 12, 1999

I can walk up to three miles—in about an hour—on the treadmill. Before the stroke, I could do about five miles, so I have more work ahead of me.

My mouth felt stalled when I talked,. but I'm trying to enjoy the pursuit of speaking again. Writing this book is part of my healing process, and often it consoles me.

July 13, 1999

Another hour of exercise while I said a huge number of words. I will be seeing my son Mark tomorrow, and I am excited about that. I haven't seen him for a year, even though he called me every day after the stroke. Eric is driving him up from Boston where he was on business. I want to tell Mark how much his phone calls meant to me. He is such a good person. I want to hug him in person.

July 14, 1999

It's a BIG deal to me.

Donna told me that I need to work more on saying multisyllable words by breaking them down into syllables. I was getting sloppy. That meant I have to go back to working with the blocks again. Donna said that the blocks were not a big deal. My retort to that was, "It is a big deal to me." She said the work was a little stone in my path. To me, it felt like a boulder! Donna said that the expression on my face was as if my best friend had died. This seemed to me to be a setback, and it was unbearably sad to me.

I understand that Donna has to push me, but knowing that doesn't make the work any easier. I half-heartedly joked that I'm paying her to be mean to me. My words sounded familiar. Once, a woman I was helping through labor said the same thing to me. I told her that I wasn't being mean, just helping her go where she wanted. I knew that she could give birth to her baby without drugs or an operation, even though her first baby had been born by Cesarean section. The woman went on to give birth to her baby just as she had planned. The memory of the woman and her words gave me hope, for I knew that Donna believed in me even when I was having trouble believing in myself.

July 15, 1999

A lesson in patience

My leg still hurts, but it seems to have more feeling in it. The massage last week helped.

In the grand scheme of things, this year in my life was a small blip. It taught me more about patience than I ever wanted to know. It caused a sudden shift in my perspective and in how I see the world.

I cry often. There is a wellspring of sadness in the depths of my soul. My psyche is fragile, and it is important to me to be surrounded by people who believe in me and in my ability to overcome this adversity.

July 16, 1999

Every day is my best day; this is my life;
I'm not going to have this moment again.
Bernie Siegel, MD

I loved seeing my son even though his visit lasted less than two days. We didn't go anywhere; we just sat and talked. Having him in the house was enough for me. I made mental pictures of him all the time he was here because I won't see him again until his brother's wedding in November.

Mark asked me to cook a pasta and ground beef casserole that he liked. I was able to cook it, and for the few minutes that the preparation took, I forgot about the stroke. I was just cooking one of my son's favorite dishes. It was an ordinary thing to do, but in my life for the past ten months, there have been few ordinary moments.

Having the stroke makes a visit sweeter. Life is so fragile—you don't know if this might be the last time you see someone.

I wish that I could put my head around a corner and see my words appear. I want to set fire to the apraxia that invaded my life and watch the malady disappear in flames. The change in my life is so profound that I sometimes can't absorb the enormity of it.

I realized that I listen better now because the aphasia sometimes forces me to be silent. I used to be like most people in a conversation—thinking about what I wanted to say next instead of listening to the other person. Because of the stroke, I'm not thinking about what to say next so I listen to others more attentively.

July 18, 1999

I argued on the phone with someone at the hospital about my bill, the first argument I've had since the stroke. I was always the one in our house to settle disputes because I had a good vocabulary and good interpersonal skills. But after the stroke, by the time I could say what I wanted, the person I was arguing with had hung up. At last I had enough words at my disposal to argue with. It helped that I felt passionate about the topic.

I didn't foresee the kind of rage that aphasia could arouse. I would get so frustrated and angry trying to say a word that I would cry and stomp around the house. Then I usually would give up and go to bed hoping that the next day would be better.

July 20, 1999

I still blunder as I try to say harder words such as "familiar" or "identifying," and I get stuck sometimes between two words that I am trying to say. I have to stop for a second and then start again. I hope all that means I am breaking new ground.

July 21, 1999

I found myself weeping again when I couldn't find the name and telephone number of someone I needed to call, and I couldn't ask Eric because he was out of town. The tears streamed down my face. I stopped crying through sheer willpower, even though I felt I could have cried forever.

July 22, 1999

I am still on a mission to get back on my public speaking "feet," but I am weary of saying, "I can do anything."

July 24, 1999

I know that I have to do day-long speeches, as that is what my clients expect, and I'm more scared than excited about it. I used to speak from notes, but now notes are not enough, so I have to write out all my speeches. First, I have to think of what I want to say. Then I have to write the speech. Then I have to rewrite the speech with the difficult words in syllables so I can say them. The emphasized syllables and words are capitalized, like this:

These pep TIDES can ALSO be found in our A mune [immune] system and are in creD a bly (incredibly) important BECAUSE they appear to MEDIATE INTER cell u lur [intercellular] Commun a KAY shun [communication] through out the BRAIN and Body.

I also use different colors or typefaces to help me know which words to accentuate or which words might give me trouble. When I'm done, a one-hour speech can be 80 pages long.

Before the stroke I could prepare a new speech in a day. Now it takes me two to three days to write a speech and two months to perfect the presentation. Sometimes the work doesn't feel worth the effort, but I must make money to pay the bills that keep pouring in. I have to quit worrying about how much I have to do and just do it.

I still can't read while the television is on in the same room. Instead I have to read in my bedroom.

Tonight my right calf felt as tight as an overtuned string on a violin. I'll be glad when the nerves are working better.

July 26, 1999

One's philosophy is not best expressed in words.
It is expressed by the choices one makes...
the process never ends until we die.
And choices we make are ultimately our responsibility.

Eleanor Roosevelt

I began the morning by saying 100 of the aphasia cards. I wanted to etch each word in my mind. I feel as if I'm an athlete training for a marathon.

I was able to wear my contact lenses for the first time since the stroke. It is a little difficult as I can't feel the lens on my finger when I put the lens in my eye and I can't feel the contact lens in my right eye.

About a month ago, Donna asked me if I thought that my writing was helping me get well. I told her it was, and now I know why. In an article about the relationship between writing and emotions, I read that when you write about a troubling event, you may feel that you are reliving it. At that point, you can change your reaction to the event by relaxing or meditating. It's like rewriting a script so it turns out the way you want it to. Writing this book has enabled me to confront my feelings and put the stroke in perspective.

Speaking is sometimes like swimming against the tide. My mind wants to say a word, but the tide forces the word back. As I was writing the book today, I wanted to complete a sentence, but one little word was missing. Little words like "at," "of," or "by" can trip me up.

I know that my brain is still healing, but I wish I had more energy. I need to keep my thoughts in the present, let my life unfold, and face problems as they arrive.

July 28, 1999

Miracles surround us at every turn if we but
sharpen our perceptions of them.

Willa Cather

I don't have curtains on my windows, so I have an unobstructed view of nature. When I sink to my lowest ebb, the picture at the window always cheers me up.

I believe that I have a better chance of speaking professionally again if I practice as many words as I can. I work out on my treadmill every day and repeat words as I walk, as if I'm walking my way to fluency. Today I felt that my persistence was paying off because I could say more words more quickly than before.

My capacity for hope is undiminished, and I draw from an inner well of faith that I will resume my career.

July 29, 1999

Kind words can be short and easy to speak,
but their echoes are truly endless.
Mother Teresa

Donna told me that I made amazing progress in the past six weeks. I don't see my progress the way she does because I am living it minute to minute. More important for me to hear than her praise, however, was her certainty that my progress would continue. I still fear that it won't.

FROM THE MASSAGE THERAPIST

When Polly was tired or stressed, she would lose concentration. She would give up more easily when she was trying to pronounce words, and her pronunciation was not as precise.

Both physical and emotional considerations are important in working with stroke survivors. Along with my desire to help Polly physically, I had a strong desire to help her emotionally. She reminded me of myself. When faced with a serious illness of my own, I became tougher. Polly was not one to be knocked down easily either, but I wanted to be there for her if she needed me.

I found that there was a tightness in her right side, and she was still numb there, so I worked on those parts longer.

Chapter Twelve
I Need a Break

August 1,1999

The only real voyage is discovery.
It consists not in seeking new landscapes
but in having new eyes.

Marcel Proust

I still wish that I could describe things deeply without so much effort. It takes what seems like forever to find adjectives and adverbs, a task I used to do in a fraction of a second.

This aphasia and apraxia are like a sliver in my soul. If I have difficulty with a new word, I have learned to stop briefly before I try to say it again. If I don't do that, I keep repeating the same sound like a phonograph needle when it is stuck.

Scott

When I talk to my mother now, I know she is no different than she was before the stroke. Her determination amazes me. For many of the tough decisions I have to make in life, I ask myself what my mother would do. She still gives me advice and makes me feel better when I am down. There are still times when speaking is frustrating for her, but when I asked her if being unable to say what she wanted to say bothered her, she replied, "Not really. You have to keep trying until you get it right." Her book will bring validation to many stroke survivors who never had the chance to express their feelings.

Brain Attack

August 2, 1999

Since we cannot change reality,
let us change the eyes that see reality.
Nikos Kazantzakis

I woke up in an introspective mood. My eyes have been opened in an incredible way, and that has made me humble. Having a stroke transformed my life. I believe that I have an obligation to tell my story so that others can realize what it's like to be aphasic. I especially want doctors, nurses, and other medical professionals to "get inside my head," so they will be able to help stroke victims more sympathetically and empathetically than if they treated only the physical aftermath of a stroke.

August 5, 1999

Alice laughed, "There's no use trying."
"One can't believe impossible things."
"I daresay you haven't had much practice." said the Queen.
"When I was your age, I always did try for a half hour a day,
Why, sometimes I've believed as many as
six impossible things before breakfast."
Lewis Carroll
Through the Looking Glass

Our trip to a doula convention in Toronto was long and exhaustive. Everybody who came to our booth told me, "You look so good and are speaking well." They were right, but they didn't have a clue how much energy I needed to be able to look and sound that way.

August 6, 1999

The terrain of the conference was familiar, but I was changed. Some of the things that people talked about seemed inconsequential to me. I was reminded of a phase I recently heard a nurse say, "I've seen life and death, and this problem is not life and death." The life-threatening brain attack altered my outlook. I feel that I redefined what is meaningful and what is picayune.

I talked so much, it felt like a kind of torture, but I did it anyway.

August 7, 1999

***History has never been dominated by the majorities,
but only by dedicated minorities
who stand unconditionally on their faith.***

R. J. Rushdoony

Seeing my friend Cheri lifted me over the hard parts of the trip. I hadn't known that she was going to be there, and I reveled in her presence. Cheri was a nurse in her 30s when she was electrocuted in a hospital elevator by pushing a button that wasn't properly insulated. Since the accident, which damaged her brain, she has been in constant pain and can't walk or write. She had to travel to the conference with an assistant and all the equipment she needed, including a motorized wheelchair. Her strength in her untenable situation was an inspiration to me. If she could be courageous, then I could be too.

Robin

The frailty I had seen in Polly six months before was gone, and the "old" Polly had re-emerged. Her speech wasn't wobbly anymore—just on the quiet side. Each word she said required intense thought, but she was confident and didn't seem to have as much difficulty finding words.

Cheri

I could see how hard Polly had been working to improve. Her gait and movements were much better than I anticipated. Her speech was much more fluent, and she didn't have to think as hard about what word she wanted to say. We talked about how she used to speak in front of groups without notes and how she now needed to see the words in front of her so she could be sure that she was saying them correctly.

August 9, 1999

The conference was draining, but at the same time, seeing so many people was rejuvenating to me. Events like these create a conundrum. Should I make the effort to do something new, or should I not take the risk? I took the risk because my determination is ingrained.

Brain Attack

August 10, 1999

Handle them carefully, for words have more power than atom bombs.
Pearl Strachan

Some people told me that travelling to Toronto was foolhardy because I was so tired afterwards. I replied that I was trying to help our finances. They told me I needed to take care of myself. That is true, but the comments were meant to wound, ending with, "If you want to kill yourself, go ahead." I wanted to tell my critics that I was trying to take care of myself and keep our creditors at bay, but I didn't explain, and I just slunk away. It was a lesson that the words I am trying so hard to recover can be used to hurt as well as to help.

August 11, 1999

Sometimes, when I start to say a word, it seems to take forever, like waiting to get to the front of a long line. You know that you'll get there, but the question is when.

I was still tired, and all I seemed to be doing was whining. Whining is all I have energy for right now. I try not to let people drag my spirit down. I can't afford to lose my optimism.

FROM THE SPEECH PATHOLOGIST

We continued to work on self-monitoring strategies for fluency and grammar correction. Polly began to write and prepare several speeches for presentation later in the summer and in the fall.

August 12, 1999

This was one of the still, hushed, ripe days when we fancy we might hear the beating of Nature's heart.
John Muir

Today was the first time since the stroke that I could feel the difference between cold and hot on my right hand. My hand itched too.

Being back at home and seeing the landscape helped me immensely. Even in the dreary days of winter, the sight of bare trees against the blue sky cheered me, I was grateful to be recuperating in Vermont where I could see such beauty every day. This must have been in the "master plan."

August 15, 1999

Never bear more than one kind of trouble at a time,
Some people bear three:
all they have had
all they have now,
and all they expect to have .
Edward Everett Hale

One of the groups for which I had been scheduled to speak this year told me they still want me to speak. I told the conference co-ordinator that her invitation showed me that people want to hear me even though I'm different. She said, "We want you any way we can get you." What a boost to my morale this was.

I got scared in the evening when I saw a small mouse. Mice don't usually bother me, but this one unleashed a high-pitched scream of sheer panic. I knew that I wasn't screaming about the mouse, but I couldn't stop screaming. My mind shut down. and I just kept making that one sound. I yelled and yelled for Eric, and when he finally came I was hysterical and was sobbing. I tried to tell him why I was so frightened. It wasn't the mouse. I had had a flashback to the brain attack—when I was yelling to Eric to save me, and no one came. I relived all the emotions that I experienced after the stroke, and it was hard to distinguish whether feelings were from seven months before or from the present. Perhaps they were all the same.

August 16, 1999

Part Therapist/Part Counselor

I told Donna about the flashback incident, and we progressed into a discussion about grief and my life before and after the stroke. I know my life will never be the same. On my down days, having Donna to talk to helps me. How do other stroke victims cope without someone to listen to their fears, worries, and dreams?

Donna gave me permission to grieve about my former life. I was working so hard to learn to talk again that I hadn't taken the time to grieve. The incident with the mouse might have been part of my grief.

August 18, 1999

...the whole of our life's experience
is but the outer expression on inner thought.
Emmet Fox

I printed a copy of my book manuscript so I could edit it during my trip to Houston to check on our house and take Eric to the doctor. Seeing the manuscript showed me how much I had progressed from being a person who couldn't spell or decide what words she wanted to say.

I was delighted to receive a letter inviting me to give one of the keynote addresses at the International Childbirth Education Association (ICEA) 2000 convention in St. Louis next August. That group was very understanding about my canceling my speeches this year. Their faith in my abilities to speak again to their audiences felt like a vindication to me. I triumphed in the moment.

I can feel most of my right hand, but my right leg still hurts.

During the flight to Houston, I read excerpts to Eric from a magazine article. I realized that I couldn't have done that as little as two months ago, and the thought gave me hope. I read to Eric often, just to practice speaking—to rewire my brain. For the same reason, I often type the same word over and over again.

August 19, 1999

Traveling was harder than it used to be. Sitting in a cramped airline seat bothered my right leg, and it hurt throughout the flight.

August 20, 1999

I spent the morning talking on the phone to friends as if I had never left Houston. I found that I could keep up my end of the conversation. Best of all, they didn't treat me any differently than before. To them I was the same old Polly. In Vermont, people don't know what I was like before the stroke.

I edited some of the book manuscript, trimming it of unnecessary words. As I did that I realized that I was writing better. My grammar seemed better too.

August 21, 1999

Today was long and grueling because I had to speak all day. Speaking off the cuff is harder than giving a speech because when I speak informally I don't know what words I'll need next. I can think of the words I want to say, but the apraxia makes it so difficult to get the words out. Talking is like trying to steer a car that's out of alignment: You have to fight to keep the car from going off the road. I fight the apraxia with motor planning, which means that to say a word, I have to think about how my mouth should be to form it. Doing that takes a great deal of effort. I was so exhausted that I went to sleep at 8:30 pm.

Ana

I spent the day with Polly. Although she still had a few pauses in her speech, it was almost as if the stroke had never happened. A woman with less fight in her would never have made the progress that Polly did.

August 24, 1999

***Although the world is full of suffering,
it is also full of the overcoming of it.***
Helen Keller

I talked for two hours with one of my doctor friends about the brain attack and its aftermath. She said that doctors need to know about the feelings I had. She asked when I was going to write a book about the stroke, and she was delighted when I told her that I had already started such a book. After the phone call, I realized that I had been "chatting." I didn't think that I would ever again be able to chat with abandon, and yet I had done it.

August 26, 1999

The trip to Houston helped me practice conversational speech. I talked day and night, and I reveled in my returning abilities. It was as if the words had been asleep in my mind, and like Rip Van Winkle they had awakened.

Brain Attack

August 28, 1999

To fear is one thing.
To let fear grab you around the tail
and swing you around is another.
Katherine Paterson

An e-mail invited me to give a two-day seminar in Iowa in April about supporting women in labor. The invitation simultaneously excited and frightened me. Could I do it? The daredevil part of me said, "sure," but the fragile and vulnerable part said, "You've lost your mind" because I will have to speak eight hours a day for two days. I'll be the only speaker. I'll have to write the speeches out and teach myself how to say them. I just have to dredge up the part of me that says, "I can do anything!"

FROM THE MASSAGE THERAPIST

While I was massaging Polly, I most noticed an extreme tightness in her right quadricep, the muscle that runs down the front of the thigh. Less noticeable was tightness in her right forearm, which seemed to restrict movement of the fingers on her right hand. I worked for longer periods of time on those areas, but I worked on the surrounding muscles too.

August 29, 1999

I exercised for 70 minutes in the morning and said some of the speech that I will give in Florida at the end of October about empowerment. Since I can't speak from notes, I had to write out the words to every one of my speeches, and I still haven't written out all of the October speech. I shuffled though such lengthy words as episiotomy [an incision near the vagina to facilitate a baby's delivery]. To say such a long word, I had to visualize it, think about how many syllables it has, and what my mouth had to do to say it.

I also said some of the words on the aphasia cards. I can say them faster, and sometimes I can do the whole card without a mistake.

In therapy I worked on percentages, but that part of my life is still troublesome to me. My homework was to write down my strategies for speaking spontaneously. There were several of them, steps people don't usually have to think about before they talk: speak slowly, enunciate, think about the first letter in the word, break hard words into syllables, look at the person I'm talking to, project my voice. I was also supposed to work on reading aloud.

I have trouble feeling safe.

August 30, 1999

More angst

This was my worst day since the brain attack. Eric's job was changed from salary to straight commission, and our income is diminishing yet again. If that wasn't bad enough, I spent two and a half hours in the hospital business office discussing my bill, which seems to be getting larger and larger. The word "huge" rang in my ears all day.

The second change in our income knocked me for a loop. In some respects, I feel that I'm responsible for our money problems. If I hadn't had the brain attack...

I am trying so hard to be able to help make a living for us. I feel so much pressure to get better before our finances get worse. I don't know if I can stay upbeat.

I have two speaking engagements in the spring, and I'm worried that I won't get the speeches done in time. I have to rewrite at least ten speeches and practice saying the words. Each speech has to be written twice—once in words and again phonetically so I can say the words. I'll write, for example, pre con seaved for preconceived, limb a ta tions for limitations, and tuff for tough. Sometimes I use different typefaces and colors to help me emphasize certain words. Often I circle a particularly difficult word.

When I think about all of the things I need to do, I feel overwhelmed. For the past seven months, I wasn't depressed, but now I am. With the financial pressures, I feel as if I have fallen into a gigantic black crater. I keep telling myself, "I can do anything," even though I don't believe it for the moment. I escape into sleep. I do like Scarlett O'Hara in *Gone with the Wind* and think about it another day.

Chapter Thirteen
Cutting the Cord

September 1, 1999

Life is an experiment.
Oliver Wendell Holmes

Today was my last day of speech therapy because it was no longer covered by insurance, and I felt as if I was cutting the umbilical cord to my womb of safety with Donna, but this has been a year of so many risks that I'm up to it.

I found out that I will be speaking again in Florida in early December to Partners in Sharing, a group I addressed two days before I had the brain attack. I doubt that my doctors and therapists would have predicted I would be talking to the same group again one year later.

I'll be paying for the effects of the stroke for the rest of my life. With our income so meager, we won't have money for things like vacations. I saw an ad in a magazine about a hotel in Maui. I'm glad I went there on a vacation 20 years ago. I'll never be able to go there again, but I have beautiful memories of it.

FROM THE SPEECH PATHOLOGIST

I have been truly amazed to reflect on the speed and depth of Polly's recovery.

September 2, 1999

I can chat once again

I took a telephone call about a business matter and realized that I must have sounded normal to the caller because he didn't mention anything. He couldn't know how I was struggling to make our fast-paced conversation seem normal.

I also got a call from a nurse about starting a doula program at her hospital. I was amazed by my ability to chat with her just as I had been when I chatted with my doctor friend a few days earlier. I talked to her for about 30 minutes before I brought up the topic of my stroke. My having had a brain attack didn't seem to bother her because she needed the information I have in my brain. When I recounted the conversation to Eric, he said, "I've been telling you that for eight months now. They need your knowledge, and they aren't bothered by the fact that you don't have perfect speech." I guess my speech deficits bother me more than they do other people.

September 3, 1999

*The Wright brothers flew right through the
smoke screen of impossibility.*
Charles Franklin Kettering

I still have a turbulent union with words. We battle for dominance. I want to set the agenda for speech, but the apraxia tries to control it instead. I'm committed to regaining all the words I used to have in my vocabulary even though they are tangled up in my mind for the moment. Words in my mind change by the time they exit my mouth. I have a few speaking engagements in the spring of next year, although the prospect of learning enough words and phrases to fill an eight-hour seminar day is daunting.

I practiced the words in the October empowerment speech as I drove with Eric to Burlington. He was calling on customers, and I wanted to go to bookstores to research books on stroke. The speech has many hard words, but I attacked them like a pit bull. I'll be speaking frankly about my drive to resume my public-speaking carreer and how I empower myself to continue working. Empowerment has become part of my mission in life.

September 6, 1999

I so love the red, orange, and yellow of fall. I inhaled Vermont's beauty— the mountains, the trees, and the forest critters.

I practiced the lecture again as I walked on the treadmill for three miles. The lecture still needs some rewriting.

I want to dislodge the apraxia from my life, but I can't. It's like an open wound.

When I listen to people saying a list of numbers, I can't remember what the first number is by the time they get to the last one, so I have to ask people to say numbers very slowly. But recently, I've been able to find the continued page in magazine articles. I remember when I couldn't finish an article that jumped to another part of a magazine because I couldn't find the page.

Robin

At first, Polly's e-mails to me were only a few words long. Now she converses at nearly the same fluency as before the stroke, and her e-mail notes are lengthy and decisive.

Polly has gone from almost constantly forgetting words and phrases to rarely having such lapses during conversations and in mail. Her spunk never left; she's just more verbose now.

September 8, 1999.

Take time every day to do something silly.
Philipa Walker

I went to sleep early last night, awoke at 2 am, and started to write in my journal. As I wrote, mountains of small postcard-size pieces of paper with my notes on them piled up around me in the bed. "What a weird to way to write a book," I thought to myself.

I wanted to write the word "gnawing," but I couldn't spell it, so I woke up Eric to tell me how. Neither of us could spell it right. I had to laugh; it reminded me of the old ad for permanent waves that asked, "Which twin has the Toni?" except it was more like, "Which of us had the stroke?" The bizarre scene was at three in the morning, and our cat, hearing the noise, came into the room meowing to be fed.

I found out that we owe about $6,000.00 to Copley Hospital. I can't figure out what to do about it. It weighs heavily on my mind and bogs me down, even when I try not to think about it.

September 9, 1999

More bad news

I thought that our financial situation couldn't get worse. Was I wrong! The situation is decomposing like a dead fish. We found out that Eric's employer will not pay any benefits, including our health insurance. I left the house in a flood of tears and walked for about two miles, crying most of the way. It's getting harder and harder to keep my spirits up.

I don't drive much because my right leg hurts every time I use the brake or accelerator. I hope that my massage session will make driving easier for me.

Brain Attack

I am still having trouble with my disability claim and the insurance authorization for speech therapy. I can't have speech therapy until I know that my insurance will pay part of the bill. My hospital bill is growing by the day. It depresses me so. The energy that I spend on these financial problems should be going instead toward speaking better and getting back to work. I don't think that these people know or care how much effort I need to explain my problems to them. Each time I call the insurance company, I have to talk to a different person and repeat my story. It seems as if the government and insurance company are trying to stall as long as they can in the hope that I'll give up. I was tempted to give up, but a friend encouraged me not to let them defeat me. She shored me up for the continued fight. It makes a monumental difference if you have people who believe in you.

September 10, 1999

A massage started my day out right, helping me endure the burning pain in my right leg. Driving was easier after the massage. I'm so grateful for my parents' gift.

My speech pathologist called me to tell me she had explained to the government office handling disability claims about my aphasia and apraxia. It helps to have good professionals in your corner. I have come to terms with the fact that there are few jobs that I could do right now, especially any that involve money because numbers are still difficult for me.

My monitrice client called me about a medical problem. This was the first time since the stroke that I needed to apply my medical knowledge. I needed a few minutes to get acclimated to the role of nurse again, but it felt good to realize that my knowledge of obstetrics was still in my head.

FROM THE MASSAGE THERAPIST

Polly reported that she was having trouble driving because her right leg hurt every time she used the brake or accelerator. When I massaged Polly, I could tell that her right quadricep was very tight, so I worked on it longer. I also used gentle stretches on her extremities.

September 11, 1999

Tentative efforts lead to tentative outcomes.

Therefore give yourself fully to your endeavors.

Decide to construct your character through excellent actions and determine to pay the price of a worthy goal.

The trials you encounter will introduce you to your strengths.

Remain steadfast...and one day you will build something that endures;

something worthy of your potential.

Epictetus – Roman Teacher and Philosopher
55-135 A.D.

At the start of every day, I have to limber up my voice. First, I have to eat, which is torture for someone like me who never liked to eat until mid-morning. Then, while I exercise on the treadmill, I read aloud the ads on the television or the names of cities on the weather map. Every cell in my body seems to pulsate with effort when I try to talk in the morning. Donna calls this "getting my mouth in gear," but I wish I could just talk in the morning instead of having to remember to warm up. I envy people who don't have to do these machinations to talk. There is no escaping the aphasia and apraxia.

September 12, 1999

I have gotten us into a really fine mess, Ollie!

I work on the October speech every day. It seems that all I do is work, exercise, eat, and sleep, and do it again the next day.

I got another unwelcome message over the weekend. I had filed an application for financial aid at Copley Hospital, and I found out that I was turned down. All that I hear seems to be the word "no." I don't know how we will pay our bills. Eric works hard and also takes care of me, and I'm afraid that our financial troubles will affect his health. I try to not worry about money, but it is on my mind night and day. Perhaps I should use denial as a way to cope.

September 13, 1999

More bad news

I started the day by exercising on the treadmill for 35 minutes.

I received four letters notifying us that the Burlington hospital had turned our account over to a collection agency .for nonpayment of bills that neither Eric nor I had ever seen. In anguish, I cried and cried.

The letters came on the heels of Eric's learning that because of the company payment schedule, he won't get any commission pay for six weeks. How will we live? I'm so frightened. This is all my fault. I have to do something to make money, but what? I'm overwhelmed with sadness, but I have no tears. Questions about our financial future fill my head, but I have no answers. I'm running out of options.

To keep my mind occupied, I worked on my October speech and its slides.

September 14, 1999

Tell me, and I'll forget.

Show me, and I may remember.

Involve me, and I'll understand.
American Indian Saying

I exercised for an hour in the morning and finished writing my October speech and choosing slides to accompany it. Now I just have to practice it a jillion times. I have only one month to get prepared.

Words engage me as they always have, and now I find that I am deriving pleasure from them as I used to.

September 15, 1999

This was a day of problems with talking on the telephone.

A customer of Eric's called him while he was out, and I offered to take a message. The caller was rude when I had to ask him to repeat his telephone number several times. As he hung up the phone, I heard an annoyed, "Geez!"

I had trouble taking the address of a woman with a confusingly thick accent who wanted me to send her a catalog. After making many mistakes spelling the words, I could tell that the women was getting frustrated with me. At last I told her that I could take the address, but I needed her to speak slowly because I had a stroke eight months ago and taking the address was very hard for me. She was patient after that.

With another order, I could tell that the woman thought I didn't understand what she was saying. Again, I had to explain about my stroke. I told her that I understood what she was saying, and the problem was in my speech and my ability to repeat numbers, not in my knowledge. She slowed down, and we finished the order better and faster. At the end of the conversation, she said, " I hope you will keep progressing."

I didn't tell the callers about the stroke until I needed to, not because I was embarrassed about it but because sometimes I don't want to waste my precious words repeating the same story over and over. I also don't like to burden strangers with the whole saga.

September 18, 1999

When I want to say something and I can't, it makes me so mad that I spit out the words ferociously

The episode of the brain attack isn't really finished, but I want to draw a curtain on that confusing time. I am learning to accept life as it is now—damaged yet enriched, poorer and, in other ways, richer. I don't see any end to the experience.

I found another magazine ad that spoke to me. It showed a family in a topiary maze, with the caption, "Life is challenging." Why is life so challenging? I'm tired of challenges.

September 19, 1999

I worked on shortening the October speech, and I also worked on the book.

Late at night my mind runs away with itself. I don't want to talk with Eric about our finances, as I'm worried that he could have another heart attack. His first one happened right after a huge financial crisis five years ago. I don't think I could bear the thought that I caused something to happen to him. I'm worried about how we will pay for his diabetes and heart medication when our insurance runs out in three months.

I have to be encouraging, but I haven't been very good about it even though I know Eric is doing the best he can.

September 20, 1999

When I put on my sneakers to exercise in the morning, I realized that I didn't have to think about it first. Previously I had to see both shoes together to figure out which was right and which was left. It was an epiphany.

I said the revised empowerment speech while I walked for an hour. I still use every second of the day in the pursuit of speaking fluently again. I continue to struggle to rebuild my credibility as a public speaker. I know that many people are unaware that I can work again. Part of my job is to remain visible on the health-care scene so that people don't shove my brochure into the back of their file.

September 21, 1999

I exercised for an hour while practicing the labor-support speech.
I finished cross-stitching a baby present.

When we were in Houston last month, the doctor said Eric would need another stress test when we went back to Texas in November for Bryan's wedding. The test will cost about $1000. I'm so scared that something bad could happen to Eric. Haven't enough bad things happened to us this year?

September 22, 1999

I exercised for 50 minutes and repeated the labor support-speech. I started correcting the grammatical errors in my book, and I could see that my grammar had improved. I don't have so much trouble with the little words as I used to. This is progress.

September 23, 1999

The ombudsman for Vermont Health Care called to tell me that she had been negotiating with Eric's former employer in Houston and the insurance company to pay more money for my hospitalization. Eric had lost his job through down-sizing, which prompted our move to Vermont. We had kept the insurance, but there was a problem between his company and the insurance company. The ombudsman thought the insurers would pay us a little more money.

A letter from Social Security about my disability application said I'm required to be examined by a different neurologist. Do the Social Security people think I'm faking? No one wants more than I do for me to be as I was before the brain attack: a dynamic woman who made her living speaking to medical professionals, not a person who still has trouble understanding what people say and has difficulty with math concepts. I asked Jane and Donna to go to the new neurologist with me. I want them to speak the doctor's language and explain what has happened to me since the stroke.

September 24, 1999

Great thoughts speak only to the thoughtful mind.
But great actions speak to all mankind.
Emily P. Bissell

A friend took me to a girls' night out to celebrate her new job. We had a lovely dinner, and I contributed to the conversation. I had a flashback to eight months earlier, when I couldn't speak at all, when my speech therapist's evaluation reported that my attempts to speak were only two words long.

Again I realized that I listen to people in a different way than I did before the brain attack.

September 25, 1999

I awoke in the middle of the night again. My sleep – wake cycles are still odd.

Today had the feeling of fall, the sun was bright, and the colors on the trees were more vibrant. I tried to change some things on our web site, but the task was very hard.

September 26, 1999

I got up early again and read. I worked on designing a flier for a new book we're selling.

My right leg still hurts, and I will go for a massage tomorrow. I have only a few massages left on my gift certificate.

I cooked supper tonight and that was a rarity, not because cooking is difficult but because eating is not important to me. Eric is usually the cook.

September 27, 1999

I started writing an article about the relationship between recovering from a stroke and giving birth, both of which require patience, strength, perseverance, courage, and determination. The article will describe how important an advocate, an empathetic doctor, and visualization are to both processes, even though birth and stroke seem so unrelated.

FROM THE MASSAGE THERAPIST

Some sensation is returning to Polly's right leg as the nerves began to regenerate and grow. Unfortunately, the sensations are burning, aching nerve pain

September 28, 1999

I spent the day talking to the medical center financial office about my bills. It took many calls to find someone who knew enough to help me. After listening to my situation, they told me they would send me a form to request a reduction in my bill. I think their answer will be "No" but I'll fill out the form. Then they'll tell me, "no."

I talked to the nurse in the office of Eric's cardiologist, and she promised to check on financial aid programs from drug companies. She is also sending me sample sizes of Eric's prescription medication. It was a pleasure to talk to a person who really wanted to help.

I feel bad telling people about my financial woes, but I need to tell someone. I guess that is what friends are for. I would go crazy without them.

Jane treated me to dinner and to a movie. I never go anywhere anymore mainly because I don't want to spend the money. There was a lot of fog on the drive home, and it scared me. I had to talk to myself to get home. Maybe I shouldn't drive at night for now.

September 29,1999

When a midwife friend consulted me about a professional problem she was having, I talked to her for about 15 minutes until I had difficulty pronouncing a multisyllable word. The mispronunciation seemed so glaring to me that I told her why the word had given me trouble. Until then she didn't realize that I had had a stroke. It must no longer be so evident in my speech.

I went with my monitrice client to her childbirth class in the evening. The night was a perfect example of the lability of a stroke victim's emotions. While I was watching the childbirth educator, I doubted that I would ever be able to teach again because my perfectionist self couldn't accept my mistakes. Eric keeps telling me that people want my knowledge, and they don't care if I make mistakes in speaking. The problem is that I care. But after the class, I decided that I could teach again, and I was certain that I would. Within a short time, I had felt both vulnerable and capable.

September 30,1999

In the evening I taught a childbirth education class to Debbie and Dale about hospital procedures and politics. My knowledge was unaffected by the stroke, and I could explain all the obstetrical information they needed. But I still had trouble with six-syllable words. I would start the word, but I always got stopped in the middle, and I found myself substituting easier words.

I hadn't been going to speech therapy, but I found out that the insurance decided to pay for my speech therapy for one more month. They never explained why. It didn't matter anyway.

Chapter Fourteen
Trying to Be a Nurse Again

October 1, 1999

People may not remember exactly what you did,
Or what you said,
But they will always remember how you made them feel.

I didn't have much to eat for breakfast, and I found myself crying as I listened to a song on a record, "Sweet Woman" by Cris Williamson. My tears were a combination of not eating and the wistfulness of the song. The afternoon went better, and my emotions seemed stabilized.

Practice will get you where you want to go, so I spent the whole day editing and practicing my empowerment speech and choosing slides for it. I competed with myself to see if I could say the speech better than the day before.

I had a session with Donna and practiced the speech some more. She told me she thought I had progressed since our previous session. Working with her keeps my spirits up, because she believes in me. I'm sure I could get better faster with more therapy, but I can't get it without insurance coverage.

I told Donna that I had been trying to remember a sentence I used to say in a speech, but I couldn't recover the words. The sentence describes why sitting on a large physical therapy ball helps women cope with the pain of labor, and I wanted to be able to use it in another speech. Donna suggested I listen to a tape of a speech I made two years ago. Eureka! The sentence was there, and I practiced it: "It elicits spontaneous, non-habituating movement." It means that unlike some methods of treating pain, which gradually stop working because the body gets accustomed, or habituated, to them, birthing balls keep working because the mother-to-be continually moves her body in order to stay balanced as she sits on the ball. Finding the sentence was a defining moment to me because it put me closer to being able to work again.

October 2, 1999

Believe in the future.

Seeing the sun rise was like a celebration of being alive. The early morning landscape that I saw through my office window was alive with color.

I cleaned the office in the morning and helped get some orders out. A hospital called to ask me to talk to them in November about a doula program they wanted to start. I wondered if I could get another speech ready in one month.

Donna has me listening to my own speeches. She thinks that will help me with my inflection and intonation. Hearing myself was like listening to an old friend. I thought that hearing my voice might make me sad, but instead it reminded me that I had been very good at my job. I vowed to be very good again, and I remind myself of that vow when I want to quit trying to speak publicly again.

FROM THE OCCUPATIONAL THERAPIST

Once I discharged Polly from occupational therapy, we changed roles. She became my friend and teacher and supported my husband and me throughout our pregnancy. Even though Polly had a life crammed with therapy, writing, and speaking, she found the time to guide us toward our goal of a natural, drug-free childbirth.

October 3, 1999

Fear and faith cannot live in the same house.
Marchant

I had a vivid dream early in the morning. I was working at a birth with my friend, took a trip to Kansas City where I'd been ten years before, ruined my clothes in a restaurant, and got a new job. It upset me so that I got out of bed, but I couldn't figure it out except that I wanted so much to work in birth again.

I exercised for an hour in the morning and practiced the labor-support speech. Only three weeks before the Florida speech, and I didn't feel ready. I was anxious about that speech and also about the doula speech I was asked to give in November. I didn't know if I could get ready in so short a time. I wasn't sure I could take that next step to recovery.

I listened to the speech that I gave in 1998 on labor-support strategies as Donna suggested. Imitating words after hearing myself say them was easier than saying them alone.

While petting my cat, I realized that for the first time since the brain attack I could feel her fur with my right hand. I luxuriated in feeling the texture of it—soft, fine, and silky.

When I get up from a chair, the right side of my body feels old and stiff, but my left side feels young. I have to hold on to the wall when I go down the stairs since there's no railing. I wonder if this will get better, but it isn't anything that is earth shaking.

October 4, 1999

Listen to the voice of nature for it holds treasures for you.
A Huron Proverb

When I got up in the morning, snow had blanketed the fallen leaves. My exercise was halted when the power went off abruptly .

The case worker for my disability claim called me in the morning. I tried to explain that I would rather work than receive disability payments but that full-time gainful employment was a long way off. I couldn't even work at McDonald's because numbers are still an enigma to me.

It has been almost ten months since the thunderbolt through my brain. I'm working feverishly trying to get well. Days go by in a blur of work sometimes. I wouldn't have described my time that way until recently because I had been doing so much repetitive work that the days went slowly. Now I feel I'm getting a handle on speaking again.

The day finished with my worrying about what will happen to us in a month or two when we have no insurance. I don't know how our life has gone downhill so rapidly. I cried softly so I wouldn't disturb Eric or cause him any more stress.

Brain Attack

October 5, 1999

You can't understand light until you understand darkness.

I went to the dentist and came away humiliated. Before I went, I asked about insurance coverage and I was told my insurance would cover my visit. They took x-rays but wouldn't fill my tooth unless I gave them $100 right away, because my insurance wouldn't cover the filling. I was honest about our financial situation and told them I would pay in installments, but they said I had to pay on the spot. I left in tears. My guess is that they did the x-rays only because they knew the insurance would pay for them. I was so upset that I couldn't eat dinner.

October 6, 1999

Just the facts, Ma'am.

I awoke feeling sad. Our financial situation blankets my days with gloom and hopelessness.

I went to Burlington for a meeting about my disability claim. I hate having to focus on what I can't do instead of on what I can do. I know that's part of the game, but it makes me feel so impotent and useless. Jane and Donna went with me, and I was grateful for their support. The neurologist was pretentious. He asked me, "How did you feel when you were having the stroke?" As I was telling him that I noticed my hearing had diminished and I couldn't turn off the treadmill, he interrupted me with, "You want to tell me the episode your way, but you need to tell it the way I want it told." I think he wanted me to talk faster and get out of his office, but I couldn't speak any faster.

I wondered if he had any information about my case. When I said that I had had tPA, he was surprised, which confirmed my suspicion that he either had no information about me or hadn't read it. I tried to do what he wanted, but in a few minutes he asked Jane and Donna, "Can you shed any light on this?" He made me feel dumb. I hoped he didn't treat his regular patients that way.

The neurologist said it was good that I had had an advocate on my side when I had the stroke, because, he said, only seven percent of people who have a stroke get tPA. As he ended our meeting, I gazed into his eyes and asked him, "Why don't more people who have a stroke get tPA?" I know that one reason is that stroke victims often don't get to the hospital until after the three-hour window for getting tPA is closed. But the core of the doctor's answer was fear of being sued because of the risk of hemorrhaging from tPA. Doctors should know that patients are fearful too, but if we were educated about risks and benefits, many of us would choose to face our fear and take the drug. The last thing I said to him was, "Doesn't it make sense that if I am the one who will recover or suffer or die, then I should be the one to decide whether to accept the risks?"

Both doctors and patients need to be taught about the risks and benefits of tPA so that patients can have a choice about taking the drug. I have been a health educator for almost 35 years, and I've had to explain complex subjects such as anesthesia and prenatal testing so that my patients could make informed decisions. I know it can be done. I wonder how many people might be leading more productive lives today if their doctors had offered them the opportunity to receive tPA.

October 7, 1999

It's a very short trip.
While alive, live.
Malcolm Forbes

A customer who called this afternoon asked about my disability. I talked to her for a long time, and I was a participant in the conversation, not just a listener. Often my higgledy-piggledy speech is like an old sweater. I know that I need to get a new one, but sometimes it is just too much effort.

Tomorrow we drive to Toronto to exhibit our childbirth products at a Lamaze childbirth education convention.

October 9, 1999

Insist on yourself;
never imitate.
Every great man is unique.
Ralph Waldo Emerson

I talked for the entire day. I was in my element because I knew the information that the childbirth education professionals at the Lamaze International convention needed.

I listened to my friend Maureen lecture. She was very good, and I hoped that I would one day speak as well as she did. Eric told me that I was speaking much better than I did two months ago. I didn't have as much trouble explaining things to people.

Brain Attack

The stairs in the hotel were a problem. Using them made my right leg hurt, especially at night.

Maureen

Polly's speech was slower that usual, but few people could tell what she had been though. When she talked about a topic she felt passionate about, there was no slowing her down. In my first speaking engagement at an international conference, Polly was in the audience supporting and encouraging me. She had been through the hardest ten months of her life, but she found time to cheer on a friend.

October 10, 1999

**Because of our routines we often forget
that life is an ongoing adventure.**
Maya Angelou

I am always trying to subdue the apraxia. At the conference, when I wanted to say a difficult word, I had to visualize it, divide it into syllables, and then try to say it, all within a second or two. It felt as if I was wrestling with part of myself every time I spoke. I had trouble speaking in the morning, probably because talking non-stop for the past two days had made me so tired. But as I was leaving the conference, one of my friends told me that she found an amazing difference in my speech since she had last talked to me on the phone. I was delighted that others could hear my progress.

I practiced my next two speeches as we drove back to Vermont after the conference. The drive was long, and sitting in the car for eight hours made my leg hurt. When I get overtired, as I did over the weekend, everything seems so desolate, but I know that this feeling will pass.

October 11, 1999

I still can't read while the television is on. Eric was listening to the TV at night, and that forced me to choose between being with him and reading. A lousy choice to have to make. Tonight I went upstairs to read.

October 12, 1999

Success is not final, failure is not fatal.
It is the courage to continue that counts.
Sir Winston Churchill

I read aloud for some time in the evening. I realized that I read faster, more easily, and with less mispronunciation than before, and I did it at night, when I typically have difficulty concentrating.

This week I read a book for only the second time since the brain attack. I used to read a book every week, but my homework and speeches leave me little time for reading books.

October 13, 1999

Real life isn't always going to be perfect or go our way,
but the recurring acknowledgment of what is working
in our lives can help us not only to survive
but surmount our difficulties.
Sarah Ban Breathnach

I talked to one of my Houston friends for about an hour in the evening. When I started speaking, I felt rusty, but as the conversation continued, I improved. It would be better for me to have people here in Vermont to talk to. I spend many days alone and don't have the opportunity to practice speaking.

I'm having trouble floating like a leaf on the current of my life, and the money demons are wandering loose again. The financial situation scares me so much, and our future is so uncertain with Eric's heart test coming up in two weeks. I try to use denial to cope, but it doesn't work.

October 15, 1999

Panic is a sudden desertion of us,
and a going over to the enemy of our imagination.
Christian Nevel Bovee

While I was exercising on the treadmill in the morning, I had difficulty hearing for a moment. My heart was pounding. I thought I was having another stroke. I quickly yawned to clear my ears, and my hearing improved. I had to assure myself that I was all right and not again descending into the depths of Hell.

I replayed the morning of the brain attack over and over in my mind. I finished exercising without incident, but there was a nagging doubt in my mind about the possibility of my having another stroke.

MEDICAL FACTS

Of the 570,000 Americans who survive a stroke each year, approximately ten to 18 percent will have another stroke within one year. The risk of recurrence increases ten percentage points in the second and third years.

National Stroke Association

October 16, 1999

In speech therapy session, we worked on inflection. Donna said that my inflection was better, but I'm not satisfied with the monotone that still creeps into my voice. It needs more work.

October 17, 1999

People become attached to their burdens sometimes more than the burdens are attached to them.
George Bernard Shaw

Today matched my mood—dreary, drab and fearful. The air was thick and heavy. I felt as if I had been beaten up for the past ten months and I was battered, bruised, and helpless. With the stress mounting, I took a walk in the afternoon after the rain stopped. Leaves in rich red and vibrant yellow sifted gently down from the trees; the ground was carpeted with them. My body moved forward, even though my will wasn't there. The walk momentarily kept my mind off our problems.

Later at night, I raged to Eric about our situation. We had to do something about it. I was at a physical and emotional ebb, desperate in a way that I had never been before. Our worries about money were sapping my vitality. My rage will be private until the book is published.

Even though Eric and I sometimes communicate with each other loudly, underneath is the knowledge that we're in the rehab process together. We are a team, and Eric shores me up when I get down.

October 19, 1999

Endurance is one of the most difficult disciplines,
but it is to the one who endures
that the final victory comes.

Buddha

I went to Debbie's appointment with her midwife today. Discussing treatment of bacterial infection in pregnancy with the midwife, I again realized that my medical knowledge is intact. After the appointment, Debbie and I went to lunch, and I remembered how much I missed my friends in Houston. My business and my life are in my house, and I don't leave it much.

I practiced saying the revised empowerment speech with more inflection. I'm always prepared for the worst during a speech, which is when the words get tied up in a knot and come out wrong. To prevent that, I need to remember my strategies for speaking—visualize, divide into syllables, plan what my mouth must do.

October 20, 1999

As soon as you trust yourself, you will know how to live.

Johann Wolfgang von Goethe

This year I found an inner resolve and strength that I didn't know I had, but I'm tired of being strong.

Eric has had to answer the same question over and over: "What is the word that I'm missing in this sentence?" I would know what I wanted to say, but the right word was often out of my grasp a lot, and I would feel stupid and frustrated.

October 21, 1999

Kites rise highest against the wind; not with it.

Sir Winston Churchill

I decided to try a technique for solving problems that a friend of mine uses. She asks the universe for what she needs, and she believes that the universe will give it to her. I had nothing to lose, so I asked for help in solving our financial problems.

The fingers of my right hand have more feeling in them now, and they itch.

Brain Attack

I talked for about 20 minutes to a nurse who is starting a hospital doula program in Nebraska. For the first time doing business, I felt like my old self. Even though my speech wasn't flawless, I used medical jargon with more ease . She was interested in hiring me as a consultant and speaker soon, so I told her that I needed more preparation time than I used to. She said she couldn't believe from my current speech that I had been almost mute ten months before. This was music to my ears. My hard work was paying off.

The conversation was so monumental to me that I had to call a friend and tell her about it. I was happy for the rest of the afternoon.

October 22, 1999

Kindness in words creates confidence,
kindness in thinking creates profoundnesss,
kindness in giving creates love.

Lao-Tze

My speech is still full of inconsistencies. I wanted to say something to Eric in the morning and I could hear the words in my mind, but when they got to my lips, the words didn't sound right. I hate apraxia!

I called a friend today, but she obviously was busy and she terminated the conversation abruptly. Something in the tone of her voice upset me, and I reacted with copious tears and a feeling of despondency. My emotions are still fragile and delicate. Working so hard to say words, I'm very conscious of how they can heal or wound.

I feel a mounting turmoil as I fend off creditors by explaining about my stroke and Eric's job difficulties. This is humiliating for someone like me who prided herself on paying bills promptly.

October 23, 1999

Only those who risk going too far
can possibly find out how far one can go.

T.S. Eliot

I practiced the empowerment speech and a labor-support speech for Florida, and I wrote out the speech for Nebraska. Before I could practice it, I had to print it out in large type so I could easily see it on a podium. Then I tried to say all the words. I spelled phonetically the words that gave me trouble. Then I began the jillion practices.

It rained all day, and I argued with Eric about our finances.

October 24, 1999

Without investment in the pregnant woman,
she cannot invest in her child.

Reva Rubin

Debbie called at about 1 pm saying that she had been having irregular contractions all morning and her bag of waters had broken. I knew she would give birth within the day. I asked her if the baby was moving as it usually did for this time of the day, and she answered yes. That "yes" is music to my ears. I told her I would come right away. I ate quickly, put my birth ball in the car, and drove to her house.

I listened to the baby's heart beat, and it was fine, speeding up a little during a contraction as it should.

I had to examine Debbie internally to see how close she was to giving birth. I didn't think about the vaginal exam until I was doing it. That's when I remembered that I couldn't feel part of my right hand. For a second, I had to think what I was feeling, but even though the sensations were unusual, I could do the assessment. I was reminded of riding a bicycle: Once you learn, you can always do it, even after a long time without practice. I determined that Debbie's labor was progressing well and she would probably give birth within a few hours.

When her contractions were three to five minutes apart, I notified the midwife that we were going to the hospital. We arrived there at about 3:15. I started to push the button for the elevator, but Debbie just walked up the stairs.

As we walked into the birthing center, Debbie had a hard contraction and went down on her knees until it was over. I instinctively started to rub her back to help her with the pain.

Debbie wanted a water birth, which meant she would spend part of her labor in a tub of warm water. The nurses readied the tub for her, and by 3:50, with delivery nearing, Debbie went into the birthing tub with her husband. The tub is large enough for Debbie and her husband.

A few minutes later, Debbie started pushing, and at 4:41 her beautiful daughter Madison was born into her arms. I never tire of seeing a mother lift out her baby herself at the moment of birth. It's an amazing sight that I hadn't seen for at least a year. I forgot how much I missed being at a birth until I was there. I realized I am still a nurse.

Brain Attack

Marje

Watching Polly work at Debbie's birth was exciting. She gave the couple the confidence they needed to face the challenges of natural childbirth. I think the birth confirmed Polly's desire to continue supporting laboring women.

MEDICAL FACTS

Sometimes when mothers-to-be labor in a tub, their babies are born underwater and quickly brought to the surface. There is no danger to the babies because the umbilical cord still connects them to their mothers and they don't begin to breathe until they are surrounded by air.

October 25, 1999

The road to success is dotted with many tempting parking places.
Will Rogers

I did a postpartum visit for Debbie and helped her go over the events of her daughter's birth. Reviewing her labor and delivery allowed me to answer her questions and correct any misunderstandings she might have had.

I must have been tired after the birth, because in the evening I was having difficulty reading. By the time I read to the end of a sentence, the meaning had already disappeared from my mind. I cried and kept saying "I'm so tired of this." Even though I've learned ways to overcome the apraxia, I'm still at war with words. My speech before the brain attack was a finely woven tapestry. After the stroke, the tapestry was in rags. The material was thread bare like a very old shirt. I wonder if I'll ever again be able to slip into speech like into a comfortable old shirt.

Through it all, Eric keeps my self-esteem high with his unflagging encouragement.

October 26, 1999

***Adventure is an attitude that we must apply
to the day-to-day obstacles of life.***
John Amat

I'm still reticent to speak informally with people I don't know. When I speak at a convention, I know the people there want to hear me. But in casual speech, I say just enough to get my point across, as if I have only so many words and I have to ration them.

The Florida empowerment speech is tomorrow. I want to give as good a speech as I gave in Chicago at the AWHONN convention. Once again, I challenged myself.

Eric

Sometimes Polly gets discouraged, and I have to remind her that people don't care if she mispronounces a few words. She wants to be perfect all the time, and she wouldn't be Polly if she didn't feel that way. I'm so lucky to have been with this woman all these years. She taught me to never give up.

October 28, 1999

***Optimism is essential to achievement
and is also the foundation of courage and true progress.***
Lloyd Alaxander

The stars were still out when we left for the airport early in the morning. There was a long, hectic day ahead in Florida.

I want my hard-earned words to empower health-care workers to help patients heal—to enable patients to use their energy to do great things. Ever since the stroke, healing has been my obsession.

I poured my heart into the empowerment speech that I gave in the evening, but I had trouble with some words and so the speech was not as stupendous as I wanted it to be. My words must have struck a chord in the audience, however, because I received a standing ovation. What came next was an utter surprise to me. The organization, the Childbirth Enhancement Foundation, gave me the first of what will be an annual award: the Polly Perez Empowerment Award. I was gratified and deeply touched to see my name on the award. To top it off, I was able to give an impromptu acceptance speech, my first unpracticed speech since December.

193

Chapter Fifteen
Pure Fear

November 1, 1999

Courage is a special kind of knowledge:
the knowledge of how to fear what ought to be feared
and how not to fear what ought not to be feared.
David Ben-Gurion

Eric went for his thallium stress test in Houston. For the test he was inject-ed with radioactive thallium. The thallium collected in his heart, which was photographed with a special camera when he exercised and rested. The pho-tographs show how much blood reaches the heart and which areas of the heart are receiving inadequate supplies of blood because of a blockage. I have such a sense of dread about the results, which we'll have in three days.

At dinner with five friends, I felt that I spoke fluently all evening and a lit-tle faster too.

November 2, 1999

I went to the hairdresser in the morning, and even though I had had break-fast, I had trouble communicating with her. She explained how she would color my hair, but I couldn't understand her. I felt so stupid. If Eric hadn't come to my rescue, explaining what I wanted done, my hair might have been multicolored.

November 3, 1999

I realized that I could feel my entire right hand. But I still can't read when the television is on. I wonder if that legacy of the stroke will ever diminish.

Being more fluent is like a frozen sea melting away, but I wish that my words were flowing more like oceans than like streams. I need to be fluent tomorrow to talk to the doctor about Eric's diagnosis and proposed treat-ment.

I talked with my former monitrice partner, and having worked with her for many years, I felt as if I were going home. I miss the professional stimula-tion of our talks.

Brain Attack

November 4, 1999

Anxiety and fear produce energy.
Where we focus that energy noticeably affects
the quality of our lives:
Focus on the solution, not the problem.
Walter Anderson

More bad news. My own heart skipped a beat when we found out that Eric has to have a heart catheterization on the Monday after Monica and Bryan's wedding in Austin. I was filled with a sense of foreboding. They will thread a long, flexible tube, or catheter, through a blood vessel into his heart to find where blockages are. I spent the day changing plane tickets and orders to go out as we were going to be in Texas longer than we had planned. Instead of being excited about the wedding, I was filled with dread.

This year has sucked! Just when my boat was getting back on an even keel, it's in danger of capsizing again. I'm so tired of bad things; I've had more than my share of them. I guess it could be worse. I can do anything. I can do anything. I can do anything.

My emotions fluctuate from hopefulness to fear, sadness, and despair, not the usual emotions for a wedding weekend. But I'm determined to have a good time at my first child's wedding and to put on a happy face for others.

November 5, 1999

Our doubts are traitors,
and make us lose the good we oft might win,
by fearing to attempt.
William Shakespeare

When I scratched the right side of my head, I discovered that for the first time in 11 months I could feel it.

I woke up at 5 am feeling uneasy, so I worked on the book to dispel my jitters. I used to say that if anything happened to Eric I could take care of myself, but now I'm not so confident.

My excitement at going to Bryan's wedding in Austin was tempered by the thought of what Eric had before him, but I put my worries aside for the weekend. My first-born is getting married! It will be wonderful to see all my family in one place for a festive celebration.

Jamie

When I saw Polly at the wedding, I noticed that the pace of her speech had improved. Occasionally she would ask for help pronouncing a word, but I remember thinking that if no one had told me that she had had a stroke I wouldn't have known.

November 6, 1999

Let all that you do be done in love.
I Corinthians 13:13

A glorious day for a wedding! Perfect weather, neither too hot nor too cold. My three sons hadn't been together for about three years. Seeing them all took me back to their childhoods. Such sweet memories! All the grandparents were there, except for Eric's mother who died the year before. I knew that she was smiling down on Bryan and Monica.

They had planned a unique day, and the wedding became a celebration. The ceremony was in the afternoon in a beautiful old cathedral. My sons and their father looked so handsome in their tuxedos. The bride was beautiful, and she and her bridesmaids carried bouquets of wildflowers.

In the two hours between the ceremony and the reception, Bryan and Monica offered their guests swing-dancing lessons. The wedding cake was topped with wildflowers, and the groom's cake was in the shape of Texas with an orange star marking Austin, where Bryan went to the University of Texas.

Dancing went on through the night. I danced slowly with my sons, my dad, and Eric. My dad danced with many of my friends and said he wasn't leaving until the last dance was done. I loved seeing him have so much fun. My memories will last a lifetime.

November 7, 1999

Should you shield the valleys from the windstorms, you would never see the beauty of their canyons.
Elisabeth Kubler-Ross

The day started badly as we discovered that Eric had lost our spending money for the trip. I sat down on the floor and cried inconsolably. As we were checking out of the hotel to return to Houston, Eric asked if anyone had turned in an envelope with money in it. They had it! And they returned the money to us when we told them what denomination the bills were.

Louise, one of my college friends, drove to Houston with us so I wouldn't have to wait for Eric's test results alone.

November 8, 1999

Valor is a gift.

***Those having it never know for sure whether
they have it till the test comes.
And those having it in one test never know for sure
if they will have it when the next test comes.***

Carl Sandburg

When we got to the hospital for the heart catheterization at 7 am, a surly woman in admitting demanded, "Where have you been?" We had a letter that told us to check in at the admitting desk at 9 am. The woman was just another example of hospital high-handedness.

After the catheterization, the cardiologist told us that Eric needed a quadruple bypass right away. My world caved in, and an overwhelming terror gripped me.

Eric's doctor had left the hospital, and I asked his partner if Eric could have the operation in Vermont. The doctor didn't try to scare me into doing what he wanted. He told us that the blockage was in a very vulnerable place, that Eric could have another heart attack, and that he probably wouldn't survive it. The cardiologist said he and Eric's doctor preferred to do the operation in Houston, but Eric could go to Vermont if he wanted.

It was the way the doctor talked to us that made a difference. He gave his opinion and didn't try to coerce us. I have been in many medical situations where fear was used to make a patient compliant—to make the patient feel guilty if he didn't agree with the doctor. We decided to have the operation in Houston, partly because the doctors had been so honest with us and we felt safe with them and partly because I have more support there.

Before I could agree to have Eric's operation done in Houston, I needed to know that he and I would be cared for as a unit. I asked the head nurse in the ICU if I could be in the ICU when we needed—in addition to the limited visiting times—as we had done when Eric had a heart attack five years before. The nurse said my request would not be a problem. If anyone objected, we were to contact her. I knew then that the nurses were willing to bend the rules to allow a patient to be with the people who would help him feel secure. That's the essence of family-centered care.

I asked if the anesthesiologist could be one of the doctors I had worked with in obstetrics. We were in luck as my favorite anesthesiologists were on duty the next day. They assured me that one of them would give Eric his anesthesia.

I thought that most of the people in the hospital understood the concept of family-centered care until I met Eric's surgeon. I told him that the head nurse in ICU had agreed to my being in the unit and how that would help Eric and me. Instantly he told me that the arrangement was impossible. I told him repeatedly that I was a nurse and wouldn't bother the ICU nurses and that the head nurse didn't see any problem. He kept saying that it would be better for Eric if I wasn't in the ICU except at regular visiting hours. The surgeon had just met Eric, and he couldn't have any idea what Eric needed or how much safer Eric would feel if I were with him. I realized the argument wasn't about Eric but about the surgeon's need to have everything his way. Eric and I were threatening his omnipotence at a time when we needed to have a rational dialogue. As a nurse, I knew that the surgeon was not in the ICU much, and I trusted the head nurse to keep her word. She was not concerned about control.

The hospital offered no pre-operative teaching. So I taught Eric myself about what would happen to him during and after the operation. I told him not to fight the endotracheal tube—the tube in his throat—because the more he fought it the longer it would take to get it out. I told him he would have to breathe deeply to prevent postoperative pneumonia even if breathing hurt him. And I told him to get out of bed as soon as he could.

November 9, 1999

Seeds of faith are always within us;
sometimes it takes a crisis to nourish
and encourage their growth.
Susan L. Taylor

The day's events were happening too fast. The nurse who came to shave Eric's chest asked me if I wanted to do it. I deferred to her as I knew that she had had more experience recently than I had. Her question was important, however, because it showed that she was thinking about Eric and me and not about herself.

When the orderly took Eric to the operating room, I felt as if I was drowning. I asked if the anesthesiologist could come to talk to me. He came right away and realized that the Perez patient was my husband. Seeing that old

Brain Attack

friend made me feel safe. He took my hand and said, "Come with me to the holding area with your husband until he goes into the OR. You both will feel better even though he has already been given a pre-op medication. Even if he doesn't know you're there, he'll know it subconsciously, and he'll feel safer and go to sleep more easily." It would have been nice if the surgeon had thought the same way and understood how important Eric's and my feelings were. I asked if someone would notify me when Eric went on and off the heart-lung machine, or pump, (both critical times), and the anesthesiologist made sure that the nurse in the holding area would do that.

I sat in a cramped waiting room right outside the ICU. Another of my doctor friends noticed me as she was walking down the hall. She checked on the operation and told me they were just starting the incisions. She promised that she would give me another update after she completed an operation of her own. Her compassion made the waiting easier.

As I awaited word about the surgery, the tension mounted inside me. Louise stayed with me, and I listened to relaxation music on my Walkman to keep my anxieties in check. I thought that after the hospitalization, Eric would face the daunting task of changing his diet and paying attention to his diabetes. I had a job in front of me too—being able to communicate with the hospital staff competently and quickly. I was a little worried about the "quickly" part. We both had scary days ahead of us.

The OR nurse came to tell me that Eric was on the pump. Three of my Houston friends arrived, and they kept me so busy talking that I didn't have time to worry. The nurse who helped with Eric's catherization reported that Eric was off the pump, and his heart was beating well. Eric's time on the pump was not excessive, so I guessed there had been no complications. The nurse had been helpful when we had to decide where to do the operation. The nurses really cared about the patient's and family's feelings.

When the surgeon came to talk to me after the surgery, he spouted a stream of information as if by rote. He spoke too quickly for me to understand. I asked him a question about the pump time, but he just kept babbling and didn't answer. Then he left. I wondered if he even knew what he was saying or if he recited something like a pre-recorded message to all his patients' families. Probably the latter, because when I asked my question, he got flustered as if he had lost his place in a recitation. My friends said they couldn't understand him either.

When I saw Eric in the ICU ten minutes later, he was awake and looked good. I was able to go into the ICU just as the nurse had promised I would. The cardiologist, anaesthesiologist, and another obstetrician friend checked on Eric, and all told me that his condition was excellent. Their visits conveyed care and concern. The nurses were outstanding about telling me what was going on. The more information I got from the doctors and nurses, the more at ease I felt.

It was nearly midnight, and the surgeon hadn't returned to talk to me since the end of the operation at noon. He knew that I needed more information than the average wife because I had told him I was a nurse. I gave him the benefit of the doubt by telling myself that he was doing other operations. While I was in the ICU waiting room, I saw the partner of Eric's surgeon talk to his patients' families several times. Our surgeon may have been busy, but I believe he needed to learn to communicate better.

I suspected he might have been almost punishing me because I asked him too many questions. In my years in the medical field, I've seen that if you challenge a nurse or doctor who needs to be in control, he or she assumes an attitude of "watch what you get now," very similar to the way the nurse treated me in Burlington when I had the stroke. All I had asked for was family-centered care. He never did return.

The other surgeon was in the ICU, when his patient's wife asked if she could spend the night. He recounted a lesson he had learned early in his medical career. He had told a woman that she didn't need to be in the ICU all the time, and her husband died before she returned. So his answer to the wife was, "You do what you feel is right."

I slept on the floor of the ICU waiting room. The hospital didn't have couches I could sleep on, and the four chairs there were connected at the arms so I couldn't rearrange them into a bed. They want patients' families to leave at night, so they make it as difficult as they can for them to stay.

Dealing with the ICU is hard for anyone but especially for a stroke victim. Speaking to people in the hospital when I had aphasia was like being in a pressure cooker. My words were slow to pop open, and I had to force them to boil and bubble up. Communicating took a huge amount of effort on my part. I had to concentrate so hard to speak quickly that it gave me a "brain drain."

The day has felt like an intense theater of life-or-death. I felt isolated even though there were people around me.

Brain Attack

November 10, 1999

*You gain strength, courage, and confidence by every experience
in which you really stop to look fear in the face.*
Eleanor Roosevelt

Eric's night nurse treated Eric and me like individuals. He volunteered information instead of just answering our questions, explained everything he was doing, and treated me like a colleague. This is what a good nurse is—part educator, part counselor, and part clinician. He also told me I could sit on Eric's bed even though one of the other nurses had reprimanded me for doing that.

The obstetrical nurses with whom I used to work offered to let me sleep in a bed in the obstetrics department for part of the night. Eric's night nurse said he would call me when he did Eric's early morning care.

I hope that in the morning they will remove the endotracheal tube from Eric's throat so he can talk and be more comfortable. I desperately want Eric to have a second chance at life.

November 11, 1999

Compassion is the basis of all morality.
Arthur Schopenhauer

I'd been told that Eric's surgeon was excellent, but he had so much to learn to be able to communicate with patients. His partner made patients feel they were part of a team. There is more to being a good surgeon than being skilled with a knife.

The cardiologist talked to us about the ventricular fibrillation that Eric was having. The ventricles of his heart were beating out of synchrony—a life-threatening problem. The cardiologist was caring and never seemed to be in a hurry even though he had a busy practice. If Eric's heart rhythm isn't normal by the morning, they will have to shock it. This was scary to me, and I went out of the ICU to call some friends for moral support. Since there were no pay phones on the floor, I went back into the ICU to use the phone there.

Then I called my office for messages. As I was returning my last call, a woman who sat at the entrance to the ICU planted herself in front of me and said, "You can't make business calls on this phone" even though I knew other people had done so. I tried to explain that I had to make business calls so I could keep our business running and pay for Eric's hospitalization.

I told her I had been on the phone only ten minutes. She called me a liar and said, "This is my area, and I'll run it how I want to." I said that I had enough stress, and she was making it worse. I was so upset that I had to call one of my friends to be with me. I can't understand why someone working in an ICU would want to make things harder for family members. I went into the hall to get away from her, and the tears in my throat came spilling out like a waterfall. When I could compose myself, I went to labor and delivery and asked if I could use their phone. They told me I could use their phone any time.

I asked for Eric to have the same nurse he had had the night before. He was smart and compassionate. The nurses in the ICU seemed dedicated to "family-centered care."

November 13, 1999

Nothing is an unmixed blessing.
Horace

The ICU nurse told me she thought that Eric was ready to be discharged from the ICU to the cardiac-care floor. Eric's surgeon's partner said that Eric might go to the floor in the evening, and we were excited about that. Our excitement was short-lived, however, as Eric's surgeon said Eric wasn't to go to the floor until the next day. I told doctor number two what doctor number one had said, and I asked if Eric's condition had changed. The doctor replied that perhaps the other doctor would come and let Eric go. He exited with, "Just watch the sports games tonight and go up in the morning," a statement that seemed selfish, demeaning, and ridiculous to me when there seemed to be no good reason for Eric to stay in the ICU. Eric and I wanted to know the doctor's reasons for keeping Eric in the ICU, but he wasn't going to tell us. He only said he would talk to us later in the day. I asked the nurses why Eric had to stay, but they didn't have a clue either. I think there must be a feeling person inside the surgeon's body, but for some reason he is trying hard to cover that up.

Our friends Nancy and Peter visited and offered to let us stay at their house when Eric is released from the hospital. That was a kind gesture, although I feel that we never will get out of here.

Later I saw doctor number two come into the ICU, but he didn't talk to us again. By 6 pm, no one had talked to us. This must have been the surgeon's way of saying no to Eric's discharge from the ICU, but no one had the courtesy to tell us so.

The extra 12 hours in the ICU probably meant nothing to the doctors, but the cost made a big difference to us. It's just another bill that we won't be able to pay. Someone should have talked to us again and explained the medical problem if there was one. Do any of these people know how much this costs? Or do they care?

November 14, 1999

Out of chaos comes the dance of balance.
Denise Kester

By 10 am, no doctors had seen Eric.

In the morning Eric said to me, "Thanks for taking such good care of me. I'd be scared if you weren't here all of the time. You make me feel safe." The nurse part of me knows that feeling safe is a big part of healing.

Like most surgery patients, Eric needed respiratory therapy to prevent pneumonia from developing in his lungs. The respiratory therapists were very good. One laughed and joked with Eric every time she came in.

Although we'd been in the hospital for five days, we hadn't seen anyone on the cardiac rehabilitation team, who should have told Eric what he needed to do to help his recovery. I taught him the post-op rehab myself with the help of the ICU nurses—diet, exercise, and the care of his incision. I guess we were the rehab team.

We left the ICU in the afternoon.

November 15, 1999

Eric was told to walk laps around the floor of the cardiac unit so he could be discharged the next day. So the day consisted of walks around the floor.

November 16, 1999

The important thing is not to stop questioning.
Albert Einstein

Anxiety abounded today. I was so afraid that something would happen to delay Eric's discharge. Both of us badly wanted to leave the hospital. The words of doctors are potent and can help us toward recovery or snatch our hope away. Then it happened. The surgeon breezed in and told us that we couldn't go home. When we asked why, he said the nurse had to change Eric's bandages on Eric's leg where a vein had been taken to be used in the bypass.

We reminded him that I am a nurse and can change bandages. I also told him that we would be staying at the house of a friend who was a surgeon. We told him as we had previously that Eric couldn't sleep in the hospital bed. He had been sleeping in a chair since the operation, and he would get more rest in our friends' home. Then I said to the surgeon that if he needed to see Eric, we could come back. He responded, "That's not as easy for me." I saw, once again, that the issue was not his patient or the family, but himself.

I asked how much money the room would cost for another day, and he answered, "Don't worry. Your insurance is paying for it." But that wasn't true because we had to pay 20 percent of the bill. I wondered if the doctor would feel the same when he sent us his bill and expected it to be paid.

I wished that I could communicate with the surgeon better. I kept thinking that I was doing something wrong, that he must have cared more than he seemed to. I asked many nurses how they communicated with him, and they said they didn't except to get orders from him. I felt better hearing that they had been working with him for many years and hadn't found a way to have an honest dialogue with him either.

My right thigh hurt a lot, probably from sitting for long periods in small, uncomfortable chairs.

November 17, 1999

Every adversity, every failure, every heartache,

carries with it the seed of an equal or greater benefit.

Napoleon Hill

After a week in the hospital, I felt frazzled with stress and anxiety. I just wanted to leave.

I thanked one of the cardiac nurses for her compassionate care of Eric and of me. She apologized for the surgeon's inability to communicate. If not for the nurses, this whole experience would have been a nightmare for us.

As we were preparing to leave the hospital, several more nurses came to our room individually to apologize for the surgeon. I told each one that I didn't blame her and that we appreciated their efforts to remedy the situation. I wanted them to know that they had done an exemplary job.

Brain Attack

One of the administrative nurses inquired about our communication problem. Then she asked me to write a letter to the administrator of the hospital. From what she intimated, I concluded that we were not the first people to have problems with the surgeon.

Being in the hospital made speaking difficult for me, especially when I needed to speak quickly in order to get the doctors and nurses to understand what Eric needed. Speaking was hardest when the doctors' body language was telling me to hurry up. Only one of the doctors on Eric's case gave me time to get all my thoughts and observations out. My mind was sharp, but sometimes my words were not. Sometimes saying a word right determined whether other people thought I was smart or a complete idiot. I can tell when people look confused if I mispronounce a word, and they begin to speak to me as if I'm a child. Doctors, with the exception of Eric's cardiologist, often finished my sentences for me, assuming that they knew what I wanted to say. Usually they didn't, and I would have to protest, "That's not what I was trying to say." Ordinarily, I can ignore that kind of treatment, but in the hospital it made a difference in Eric's care.

One doctor treated me like a half-wit and didn't try to understand that I had medical knowledge. He must have thought, "She can't know what I'm talking about."

I worked on the book as a way to relieve my frustration. It was better to bang a pencil on the paper instead of on the people I was angry with.

We left the hospital in the afternoon and went to our friends' home. I felt so lucky to be there. I had weathered the storm.

Nancy

I met Polly for the first time when she worked closely with my husband Peter, to establish a woman's hospital in Houston. I had heard of her determination, energy, and ability to accomplish a multitude of tasks. Frequently, she was confronted by doctors resistant to change. The same character traits of persistence and endurance contributed to her incredible progress in recovering from the brain attack.

At the hospital I saw Polly become frustrated only when she had to communicate with some of the doctors who, because her speech was slow, treated her as if she wasn't very bright. She never had much patience with arrogant doctors and certainly disliked being treated as a child. Although Eric's recovery period was exhausting for her, I never noticed any loss of speaking ability, which might have been expected from someone who was physically and mentally exhausted. Her inner strength served her well once again.

November 21, 1999

Never give up.
This may be your moment for a miracle.
Greg Anderson

When the immediate post-operative period was over, I had time to reflect on the huge amount of work I needed to do to keep our business running. Our Vermont friends put part of their lives on hold, went to our office every day, and got orders out while we were in Texas, saving us many irate customers. One friend even took her new baby to our office with her.

November 22, 1999

Nature is the common, universal language understood by all.
Kathleen Raine

I had to drive in the Houston traffic for the first time since the stroke. Despite the stress, Eric said I did fine. At night I felt I had trouble processing information, as I did right after the stroke. There are so many people and so much hustle and bustle in Houston. I pined for the picturesque scenery and quiet of Vermont.

Peter

Polly had significant improvement in her motor function and verbal skills since I saw her in March. Still, I imagine Polly may never have full recovery, which is sad.

November 23, 1999

The most perfect union between spouses
is not that which they express when rejoicing together,
but that which they show when they suffer together,
one for the other, one with the other during hard times and in spite of it.
The union in joy makes the union in difficulty.
Raniero Cantalemess

During Eric's appointment with his cardiologist, the office staff was kind, and the doctor answered our questions patiently. He said that Eric was lucky to have a wife with medical knowledge. We saw the surgeon too, and for the first time he treated me as if I had a brain in my head.

We were cleared to go home. Hallelujah!

Brain Attack

November 25, 1999

Giving is the highest expression of our power.
Vivian Greene

We went home to Vermont, and the trip was like a tonic to me. Friends had Thanksgiving dinner ready in our home.

November 26, 1999

I was strong throughout the past two weeks, but in the evening I let my emotions run rampant. I'm so frightened that something I do will hurt Eric. I know that's not rational, but it's the way I feel.

November 29, 1999

I have to drive everywhere, and driving is sometimes still daunting to me. I'm always aware that a mistake could hamper the healing in Eric's chest.

Even though I speak better, I still find that words occasionally elude me. I read a book about stroke that called the year after the stroke a vacation from work. It was no vacation for me. Instead it has been an angst-ridden year of the hardest work I've ever done in my life.

From the Editor

While most people judged Polly's recovery through her speech, I saw it in her writing. As I edited her manuscript, I made the kind of triage that is well known to health-care professionals. Some of the text I left alone, some I edited for grammar or clarity, and some I deleted. The deleted text consisted primarily of repetitive passages, points that Polly had made before.

As I lived Polly's year through her writing, I gradually needed to make fewer and fewer corrections for clarity and grammar. While I had to continue to ask for definitions of medical terms and fix an oddly persistent difficulty using "a" and "an," most of the writing began to fall in the first group: leave it alone and let Polly tell her story.

Chapter Sixteen
Better Than Last Year

December 1, 1999

You can't depend on your eyes when your
imagination is out of focus.
Mark Twain

Eric listened to me say the empowerment speech in the morning before I had to give it. He's heard me practice it so many times, he could probably give the speech himself. At times I was talking almost as well as I used to, before the brain attack. When I talked as fast as I used to do, I made more mistakes, but it felt good to speak at my normal rate of speed again.

When I gave the speech, I noticed that my inflection and phrasing were better, even though I had practiced the speech for only two days. I got a standing ovation, and after the speech I answered questions for the first time since the brain attack. Answering questions is harder than giving a speech because it means speaking spontaneously—deciding on an answer and saying the words in the few seconds I have to respond. I still have to think hard to converse spontaneously.

December 6 , 1999

Words are the voices of the heart.
Confucius

We met Eric's new cardiologist and surgeon. The cardiologist was refreshingly approachable and attentive to what Eric and I said. He answered all our questions and even asked several times, "Are there any more questions I could answer for you?"

Eric's leg was swollen, and the surgeon told him to not walk for two days but to keep it elevated to relieve the swelling. For the rest of the day I cared for Eric as he lay on the couch with his leg raised, and I also sent out business orders. Once I'm caught up with orders, I have to write and practice about 12 speeches for the spring.

December 7, 1999

Never confuse a single defeat with a final defeat.
F. Scott Fitzgerald

In the morning I got a long-awaited massage, and it eased the stress I was under. My parents' gift of massages was the best I've ever received.

It's unlikely that we'll get a Christmas tree this year, as I don't think I can decorate it by myself.

I completed the application for financial assistance for the medical center hospital. I hate having to ask for financial help.

FROM THE MASSAGE THERAPIST

With so much more stress in her life since I last saw her, Polly really needed her massage. I worked on her whole body, giving special attention to her right thigh.

I'm grateful that I worked with Polly. She enabled me to face my fear of working with a challenged person, and eventually I enjoyed our time together. In the end I didn't see her as challenged or disabled. I thought that I was going to give her emotional support, but there were times when she gave emotional support to me.

December 8, 1999

Always bear in mind that your own resolution to succeed
is more important than any one thing.
Abraham Lincoln

The day was somber and grey, and my spirits matched the weather. Today all of my words came out of my mouth wrong. When that happens, it is like opening up an old wound.

I had to drive home from dinner at Jane and Michael's house after dark, and driving after dark is still scary to me. Whenever I drive, I worry that even the smallest accident could hurt Eric's chest. He won't be able to drive himself until his chest is completely healed.

December 9, 1999

*If one advances confidently in the direction of his dreams,
and endeavors to live the life which he has imagined,
he will meet with success unexpected in common hours.*
Henry David Thoreau

It's an understatement that today was better than the same day one year ago. Sometimes I feel normal, but then the apraxia surfaces and I can't say something that I want to say but my bull-headed determination surfaces and I just start trying to say the offending word again. I use these apraxia obstacles to help me focus on my long term goal of working as a public speaker. That focus is unwavering.

Passion and commitment has a way of making good things happen and I celebrated the passing of one year after the brain attack with the people who were my constants during the year: Jane, Michael, Donna, Marje, Bob, Debbie, and of course Eric.

Marje

Throughout the past year, I saw Polly overcome one obstacle only to confront another. She never gave up and became only more determined. I watched her turn her stroke into an opportunity to educate the public, health-care organizations, and health-care workers. I saw her explore why things happen and use her misfortune to help others.

December 11, 1999

*If you watch how nature deals with adversity,
continually renewing itself, you can't help but learn.*
Bernie Siegel, M.D.

I awoke with a start from a bad dream about Eric's health and our financial situation. To calm my nerves I started reading. Through my window, I saw only blackness, which changed after a while to dark blue and then to a soft light blue. Then I could see that in my backyard snow covered the Adirondack chairs where there hadn't been any snow when I went to sleep. The trees wobbled in the wind. I was so glad I live here. The quaint scene made me feel I was in a safe haven once again.

Brain Attack

In order to write a word, I have to say it first, but I still have trouble sounding out some of the words I want to write. There is no rhyme or reason to the problem. I might have trouble with "put" and "pat," when a multisyllabic word such as "anesthesiologist" gives me no trouble at all. Apraxia is like a monster hiding under the bed. You don't know when it will leap out.

December 12, 1999

Courage doesn't roar.
Sometimes it is the quiet voice at the end of the day saying,
"I will try again."

The incision in Eric's leg where the vein was taken for the bypass has a persistent infection and is not healing as it should. I try to see the positives rather than the negatives but sometimes all this seems too much for me to handle. I must remember my mantra "I can do anything."

Sue

I gave a lecture about collaboration between doctors and nurses to improve patient care to an audience consisting mostly of doctors. I emphasized that if professionals didn't work together to minimize medical errors, someday one of them could be lying in a hospital bed alone and abused. Polly's face and her words about empowerment were in my mind throughout the lecture, making me confident that I could teach the doctors in my audience. After the lecture, people told me they had never thought about the topic and they hoped they could make a difference in their practice and in their relationships with other health-care providers.

December 16, 1999

Some people see things as they are and say "Why?"
I see things that never were and say, "Why not?"
George Bernard Shaw

I saw my physical therapist and asked him if he knew when he met me a year ago that I wouldn't be a typical patient. He answered, "I knew that you would be different because you wanted to start rehab on Christmas Eve." I told him I desperately wanted to get well and didn't want to waste any time.

This journey has been about traveling outward. I have to accept the contrasts in my life. The ugliness of the stroke and the beauty of the world around me. Ferocity and tenderness. Faith and doubt. Courage and insecurity. Throughout the whole year, I was searching for my words. I realized that they were there all along, but apraxia covered them up like the snowdrifts I see from my window. With help from my therapists, family, and friends, I plowed a path back to speech. I wonder if my progress will continue.

December 17, 1999

You have to have confidence in your ability,
and then be tough enough to follow through.
Rosalynn Carter

I still can't do much with numbers, but I was trying to figure out how old Mark would be on his birthday this week. I knew that he was born in 1969, but I couldn't figure out how old he was. Tears streamed down my face because I felt so dumb not knowing how old my son was.

December 18, 1999

My life is my message.
Mahatma Gandhi

I think people who don't live with a disability can't understand how the disability gets integrated into your reality. Just when I think I can speak perfectly, the gremlin apraxia peeps around the corner snickering, "Gotcha!" Then I take a breath and start again, and he disappears. But I know he will be back. Aphasia and apraxia are part of my existence now, even though I don't like that. For life, I am a person with aphasia and apraxia. Often my words are paralyzed but my spirit is not.

How has this trip to aphasia-land changed me? I learned that as you accept your limitations you can better focus on your strengths. Aphasia taught me lessons that I wouldn't have learned otherwise, such as how it feels to have a disability and how people treat you differently when you are disabled, how some people equate not speaking well with stupidity, how important it is to really listen to what someone is saying, and how powerful words can be.

My brain attack has made my life sharper. I am acutely aware that I have a finite amount of energy and time and I choose better now when I speak. I have to ask myself if it is worth it to say things. Sometimes it is and sometimes it isn't. All words now are very precious to me.

I still have difficulty reading at night. I have to concentrate so hard to make sense of the words on the page, that I usually give up and go to bed.

December 19, 1999

Life is uncharted territory.
It reveals its story inside you.
Leo F. Buscaglia

The sleep I got at night cleared up the cobwebs in my brain, and I sat in my recliner in the morning and read. Printed words are distinct in the morning but not at night. My cat snuggled next to me as I read, and I reveled in the feel of her fur on my right hand. To me, this moment was wrapped in splendor and I reflected on the time a year ago when I couldn't say her name no matter how hard I tried.

I worked harder during the past year than I have ever worked in my life, but I was the only one who could do it—no one could do it for me. I see many similarities between my recovery and giving birth to my children, another job no one could do for me. My birth experiences showed me how tough I could be, and giving birth without drugs to dull the pain taught me that I could do anything. I'm thankful that I learned that lesson to help me face the year's trials. With an unwavering sense of purpose, I pushed through the year and learned that I could go places that I never dreamed I could go.

FROM THE MASSAGE THERAPIST

I realized that working with Polly helped my self-confidence as a practitioner, and I am flattered that she put her trust in me. God must have sent her to be my first client to suffer from the effects of a stroke. Her strength of will was amazing.

December 20, 1999

The optimist sees opportunity in every danger;
the pessimist sees danger in every opportunity .
Sir Winston Churchill

I worked all day trying to get ready to do the winter speeches and the accompanying administrative work. I feel that most of the time I am carrying an oversized burden and was I worry that I might drop it.

The bills for Eric's surgery and hospitalization are rolling in, causing an undercurrent of worry about finances again.

December 21, 1999

Joy is prayer.

Joy is strength.

Joy is love.

Joy is a net of love by which you can catch souls.

Mother Teresa

I awoke at 3 am, read, and worked on the book.

After stewing for a long time about spending money frivolously, I bought a Christmas tree at a place that sold small trees for $15. I decided that the tree would be my Christmas present. It was small enough to stand on our coffee table, and Eric and I decorated it. I so love Christmas and the message it brings to the world.

December 24, 1999

Motivation is an external, temporary high that pushes you forward.

Inspiration is a sustainable internal glow which pulls you forward.

Thomas Leonard

I was trying to write, and I was irritated to find that "brain fog" was moving in. I had to get something to eat before I could continue working. Still, I certainly feel better than I did one year ago, when my vocabulary was pared down to a few words and confusion reigned in my life. 1999 has been about the three D's: desire, discipline, and dedication.

Part of my life will remain a mystery until I can relearn my math skills. It's as if part of my life has a hole in it. I decided to ask Debbie to teach me more math, so I can calculate percentages again. I hate when I can't figure out the cost of something on sale, like 30 percent off the regular price.

December 25, 1999

I will honor Christmas in my heart and try to keep it all the year.

Charles Dickens

Christmas gave me the joy of renewal and hope for tomorrow and wrapped me in its magic. The sun shone through the pines as we went to Christmas brunch with two friends, and the day had a gala feeling to it. It was a lovely way to spend Christmas.

Brain Attack

I can feel most of my right foot except for parts of the sole, and walking is easier even when it is snowy and icy outside.

For a Christmas present, Bryan and Monica gave us enough money to pay the spring installment of our real estate taxes. It was a huge surprise and touched us so deeply. Another surprise was a gift certificate for massages from Mark and Jamie.

December 27, 1999

There is no agony like bearing an untold story inside you.
Zora Neale Hurston

I started back on my daily exercise routine, combining the treadmill with practicing speeches or multisyllable words. While I was exercising, I had another skirmish with words. Will I ever get the apraxia under control?

I spent all day working on the book. Writing this book is a way to not shield myself from the reality of being disabled. Apraxia and aphasia is like going through an odyssey every day and the trail is treacherous. Through the book, I want the reader to soak up how it feels to be disabled and what you can learn from it. I see the book as something positive that can affect others.

Next I need to work on the speech about doulas and nurses working together that I am to give in Nebraska in a few weeks. I'm a little afraid to leave Eric alone for three days when I have to work out of town.

I fret about the, unknown and the bills keep piling up. This year has been a black, black night that has gone on too long, an endurance test of unimaginable proportions. .

December 28, 1999

Everything is possible for him who believes.
Mark 9:23

When I speak or write, I don't have to grope for words as much as I used to. The words such as by, at, with, and in that I used to call little words have returned to my vocabulary. I don't know where the little words were hiding in my brain, but I'm glad to see them again.

I realized that my words no longer feel so imprisoned in the jail of my mouth. Words are mine now most of the time, but I still play a cat-and-mouse game with them. Living with aphasia and apraxia is confusing. You don't know if the next word that you say will be the right one or a mixed-up combination of syllables.

Stephanie

When I spoke to Polly, I actually forgot that she had suffered a stroke just a year before. The only trace of the stroke in her voice was the occasional pause and the "mmm" that she said when she was trying to recall an elusive word. But it was much like anyone else would say "mmm".

I'm sure her life is not exactly as it was, but the distance she has come is remarkable. I forgot to speak slowly to her. I forgot to feel sorry for her. When I hung up from the conversation, I had to fight back tears again. My friend was back from her silence.

December 29, 1999

For as he thinketh in his heart, so is he.
Proverb 23:7

I thought that we owed the Vermont hospital a lot until I saw the staggering sums that we owed for Eric's surgery in Texas. We keep getting a bill from a doctor that we don't know. I can't fathom how we can pay the bills on the small amount of money that Eric and our business make. Our insurance runs out in two days.

Eric still has a lot of pain in his right leg. I would rather be the one who is hurting.

I am so tired. The past six weeks were so draining. I have to say more affirmations about my ability to do anything.

Mavis

As a doctor, I chose Polly to be my monitrice during the birth of my two children because I wanted to be sure I would have individualized care. For her to be a nurse who had strived all of her life to support and comfort others and then to have been denied support after she had a stroke was a health-care provider's worst nightmare. Knowing Polly as I do, I was not surprised that she saw the incident as a blessing in disguise and used the experience to teach others.

ack

December 30, 1999

The most powerful weapon on earth is the human soul on fire.
Marshall Foch

I sketched out three speeches for my spring lectures. Now I have to practice saying the words in them. One of the speeches is about "intracutaneous injection of sterile water" (a way of easing the pain of so-called back labor, when the baby is facing forward instead of backward, by injecting a little water under the skin of the woman's back. The water stings, and the back pain is temporarily suspended.) If I can say just the topic of the speech, I can certainly talk better than I could a year ago.

I cried and cried in the afternoon because our insurance runs out on January 1 and we had to cancel Eric's doctor's appointment until we are able to pay for it.

December 31, 1999

How you do anything is how you do everything.
Zen Proverb

The past year was like an emotional triathlon. I'm reminded of the words of Ralph Waldo Emerson, "Patience and fortitude can conquer all things." Sometimes the year seems to have gone by in a blur; other times it was plodding. I was able to come out on the other side of misfortune. I realize that the gifts I received this year, faith, love, and hope among them, were priceless. I learned to ask for help, to build a support team around myself, and to invent creative solutions for my problems. I learned to tell time, do math, type, spell, write, speak, walk, balance, and drive. I believed in myself and my future, and I persevered, no matter what lay before me. I know that with others' love and support, I can do anything!

Mark

Some people may think that the progress my mother has made in just over a year is remarkable, but I expected it because she always told me, "You can do anything as long as you believe in yourself," and she did. That's why she is my hero.

A New Millennium

January 1, 2000

The only way through pain... is to absorb, probe,
understand exactly what it is and what it means.

To close the door on pain is to miss the chance for growth.

May Sarton *Recovering: A Journal 1978-1979*

I started the year out right, like a good Texas gal, by eating black-eyed peas to ensure good luck. Maybe that's what I was doing wrong for the past few New Years.

I spent New Year's Day doing mundane tasks, such as taking down the Christmas tree, but I reveled in being able to do them, when 12 months ago I was a shell of myself.

Chapter Seventeen
My Saints

This episode in my life unfolded like the painting of a picture. From within the shelter of people who loved me and believed in me, I created a painting, brush stroke by brush stroke. I knew that I had to do the painting myself, but I needed assistants to encourage me when I encountered a difficult segment of canvas. As they made my life better, the painting began to look more vibrant.

Eric was loyal, honest, and forgiving, and he loved me unconditionally even when I vented my frustration on him. He took to heart our marriage vows about sickness and health. Even when I wavered in my belief that I would recover, he never faltered. We had no doubt that we would get past this together.

My rehabilitation team became my extended family. My very competent therapists were my collaborators as I applied paint to the canvas of my new life. They wanted me to paint a magnificent landscape. They helped me make sense of my shattered existence. Just a few minutes of their time made me feel special and enabled me to work more effectively. They were there not to push, but to encourage gently. They gave a face to health care and helped make it more human and humane as my painting came alive.

Working with a speech therapist is one of life's most intimate and complex experiences. Donna was the key to my speaking future. I drew on her strength. What started as a tentative alliance, strengthened over a year into a working partnership of two extraordinary women. My journey with Donna began with a few tentative words, and it will end, I hope, only when my speech becomes, once again, a simple, intoxicating joy.

Steve, my physical therapist, made me laugh and helped me find new energy when I was too tired to continue exercising. Debbie, my occupational therapist, cheered toward my goal of being able to do math and tell time again. Our friendship culminated in my attending her during the birth of her daughter, Maddie.

Through the year, I kept painting. Often Jane and Michael stopped by to check on the progress of my life design and helped keep me at the easel. My parents, sons, and father-in-law often checked on the project and gave it color and shading. My friends in Texas and Vermont and on the Internet gave me a new brush when I needed one.

My repainted life holds many original, artful touches now. It's a unique portrait that I could not have created alone.

Chapter Eighteen
When we're ready to learn the lesson, the teacher will appear.

The brain attack changed my life and my soul. I was always cerebral and left-brained (analytical), but the stroke forced me to get more in touch with my right brain. I had to become more intuitive, to express myself more through gestures than through words, and to be more free with my feelings than I had been before.

As a baby learns to speak, I learned to speak again by trial and error and infinite practice. Even though my speech therapy ended ten months after the stroke, I continue to improve through constant practice. Life is my speech therapist now.

My journey to "stroke-land" was different from any journey I'd taken before, but it was worth all the effort because I learned to laugh at myself and to trust myself. Before the stroke, I wouldn't have been able to see a brain attack as an opportunity for growth, but it gave me the chance to delve deep inside myself and find I was tougher than I thought possible.

If not for the support of my family, friends, and therapists, I wouldn't have been able to recover as well as I did. For a year I devoted myself to being able to speak again and to pursuing my passion of educating health-care providers. I made up my mind that I had to heal and relearn my lost skills. I know that I have ahead of me a future full of challenges and opportunities and, I hope, many ordinary days.

I trusted that this experience was ordained to happen and was not a mistake in my life's curriculum. I had to trust that the process would help me. (If I didn't learn something by the stroke's clobbering me, I don't want to know what it would have taken to get my attention.) The experience changed my life perspective. I had been so focused on living life, that at times I didn't enjoy it. Now I take nothing for granted, not even the view from my window. I would not want to travel this road again, but if I had stayed on the same path, I would have missed new people and experiences.

In setting a course to retrieve my lost words, I found that endurance was my best friend, and consistency was my best guide. Speech therapy is the hope for my fellow aphasics and me. I fought unceasingly to make my mouth say the words that my brain sent to it. I practiced talking day and night, but I wished sometimes that I could reach my goal of speaking fluently by skipping ahead or racing. But the only way for me to reach my goal was by plodding along one step at a time.

My moods were intense and seesawed wildly. I produced a symphony of cries, groans, screams, yells, shrieks, and howls that I wouldn't have thought was possible. I don't remember ever making those sounds before, but they helped me express what I was going through. I cried more that any other time in my life. Later in the year, my sounds were mixed with laughter and glee as I felt better about myself and my life. All the sounds were important to my healing.

Writing a book for people you will never meet is a way to share something that is important to you. I wrote this book to put my experiences into words that would help others. At the same time, the writing and its intimate reflections were a form of grieving for my pre-stroke life and a kind of psychological therapy. Writing each day gave me a new perspective on what was happening to me, like a photographer pointing a camera in a different direction. The result was a picture of my life as I had never seen it before.

I have written about loneliness, fear, anticipation, frustration, and fulfillment. I am no longer the person I was before the brain attack. The book helped me find a voice when my speaking voice was temporarily silent. Since I couldn't write or spell after the stroke, writing the book has been a great achievement for me.

Writing changed my relationship to the trauma of the stroke, and it helped me handle an arduous time in my life. It was a way to console myself. The writer Alice Walker has described writing as "a very sturdy ladder out of a pit." The year after the stroke often felt to me like a bottomless pit, and to paraphrase Walker, I wrote to save my life.

Patients as well as health-care workers can use writing to express their feelings. Writing helps us discover where we have been, see where we are, and understand where we are going. Writing a journal during the year after a stroke—or after any traumatic event—helps the writer appreciate what new doors in life will be opened by the disability, even as some doors may be closing.

When I finished writing the book and entrusted my hard-fought words to the editor, I felt a certain foreboding. What had I done? I had let the whole world know my innermost fears, thoughts, and dreams. But I researched the information that had been published about strokes, and I found that little had been written about the feelings of patients recovering from a brain attack. Perhaps the feelings were too painful to write about. That's when I knew that I needed to make my private thoughts public in order to help others going through the kind of trial I faced and overcame.

Things do not change, we change.
Henry David Thoreau

As painful as my loss of words was, it reminded me of the old Australian tradition called a "walk about," a time to take a break from work to go on a long, contemplative, solitary walk and return revitalized and clear eyed. On my particular walk about, I learned many lessons. I realized that I didn't have time for small problems. I learned that I could be sad and still be hopeful too. I recognized the importance of taking risks. I understood the challenge and the meaning of survival. I acquired a tremendous reverence for the power of life.

Things I learned from my struggle

You can find a ray of light in the darkest cloud.

You must listen to your inner voice.

You can turn a negative into a positive.

You shouldn't give up when you still have something to give.

Endurance is your best friend.

Nothing is over until the moment you stop trying.

A sense of humor, hugs, and laughter do wonders to counteract the stress of frustration.

Trust your feelings and make your own judgements.

Give yourself the gift of time.

Persevere and work hard to attain your goals and dreams.

Have faith in yourself.

Having a stroke is not the first thing to do in a new town, but it is an innovative way to meet people.

Never stop looking for things that challenge you.

Life can be terrifying, and it can be beautiful too.

If one door closes, another one opens.

Never give up the fight.

Nothing is tougher than you are.

Brain Attack

The day I had the stroke began as an ordinary day. The day I write this is another ordinary day, but a day like this is such a little miracle to me now. I feel gratitude for this day of wonder—an "ordinary" moment in my life. I am on my own now, and humor and faith sustain me. Life is a constant challenge, and I'm eager to see how the next chapter unfolds. I hold onto normalcy as if it is a life preserver.

I hope that this day and the next and the next are, in most respects, normal....

The end of the thing is never the end,

something is always born..

Lucille Clifton

Part II

Revamping Attitudes toward Health Care, From a Nurse's Perspective

Some people thought that I was making a mistake by doing my rehabilitation in a small hospital, but one of the things that made Copley unique was its emphasis on personally knowing the patients and their family and friends.

The therapists I had at Copley—Debbie, Donna, and Steve—gave me part of my life back. I felt supported and unjudged by them as they helped me stretch and grow. The strength that I needed was inside me, but sometimes I needed help in finding it. I exposed vulnerability and trusted them, and they trusted me. Their trust in me fostered my healing.

The Copley staff's mastery of emotional support and personalized medicine stood in contrast to my treatment at the medical center in Burlington. At the core of that awful incident was the nurses' lack of caring. On the ward, the nurses viewed their patients as the enemy.

The only power issue that should concern health-care professionals is the power of caring and deep respect for other people. From my experiences as a nurse and then as a patient, I realize that medical professionals should tell patients what the patients can do instead of what they can't do.

I know that under the pressure for changes in the health-care system, nurses are caught in a downward spiral of insufficient resources and personnel and in outmoded roles. But laughing at me when I couldn't speak and needed the nurses' help was not about being overworked but about power and control. There was an imbalance of power, which impairs the building of a solid relationship between the patient and health-care workers. Instead of struggling for power, we in health care should be honest with our patients about how we make decisions and then we should make decisions with our patients, not for them. Patients should be able to decide what risks they can comfortably accept, instead of accepting the risks their care providers are comfortable with. Patients need to share the responsibility for decisions about their medical care. If that happens, health-caregivers won't feel so fearful and in need of defending themselves.

God protect me from self-interest masquerading
as moral principle.

Mark Twain

Mergers and managed care have changed health care in many ways. Because mergers are about containing costs, they often provide no benefit to the patient while raising enormous potential for conflicts of interest. What's wrong with this picture is that patients become invisible.

Unlike corporate enterprises, healing should be a human interchange where the power of intimacy dominates. But right now, intimacy in health care has been replaced by a series of political fights between those who manage the business of care and those who want to provide healing. We seem to have let technology and materialism take the place of caring with no one representing patients' interests.

Attending to patients' emotions takes time, of which health-care workers are in short supply. Lack of time has forced professionals to abandon the magic in health care. To recover it, we need to take the time to create a relaxed atmosphere and talk with our patients. If we do that, we will hear an expanse of emotions, including fear, anger, despair, and frustration. Perhaps that is why we don't talk to our patients: We're afraid of what we will hear. Instead, we should let our compassion and sense of humor show more. We must not punish either patients or professionals who work by "coloring outside the lines." We should be willing to seek advice when we don't have an answer. We must approach routine tasks in new and creative ways, such as reconsidering restrictions on family visits and making families part of the caregiving team.

No problem can be solved from the same
consciousness that created it.
We must learn to see the world anew.

Albert Einstein

Change brings challenges and responsibilities, but altering habitual behavior is difficult. We must let go of old practice patterns and leadership styles if they aren't empowering patients to heal themselves. We should look at our policies through the eyes of our patients and ask, "What do our patients want and need?" "How do they feel?" Instead, we sometimes act like benevolent dictators who know what patients need, even if they disagree.

Our bodies are where we stay. Our souls are what we are.
Cecil Baxter

Compassion and caring are essential in patient-care relationships. We must put humanism first. Although bonds in health care are not easily formed, once broken, they are even more difficult to rebuild. But in order for our patients to trust us, we must trust them. Trust is a two-way street, and it forms when everyone in a relationship is equal. The most productive change in patient and caregiver relationships is likely to occur when patients, physicians, nurses, and corporate managers step outside their narrowly defined positions and begin working together, talking to one another, and respecting one another's feelings and opinions.

We need to provide an environment where patients can heal. We must invest not just our lives but also our hearts. We must give voices to those who have none and teach our patients to have courage. We must understand the anger and frustration that stroke victims sometimes feel.

If we like ourselves, we usually have a good relationship with our patients. We must be responsible for our own behaviors and help our patients to be responsible for theirs, or we will be in a permanent state of suspicion and warfare. Health care is not supposed to be adversarial. We will make more progress if we work together. We must go beyond competition to cooperation. We must respect one another's strengths, compensate for each other's limitations, and recognize our interdependence. We should be kinder to one another. It's amazing how powerful "hello," "please," and "thank you" can be in a relationship.

I was privileged to work with professionals who brought a spirit of collaboration not confrontation to their work with patients. From my rocky start, I would never have thought that the elements in my recovery would come together in an unbelievable way. That coming together is called synchronicity, and patients reap the benefit of it.

As we work through the changes in medicine, we have to make flexibility a key concept in our care. We should be courageous enough to examine our practices from every angle. We should not be afraid to change directions or to be creative. Our patients are depending on us.

We must always change, renew, rejuvenate ourselves;
otherwise we harden.
Goethe

Attitudes Toward Health Care From a Patient's Perspective

Those of us who have had a stroke or other brain injuries want to have the opportunity to prove ourselves and remain productive members of society. We need health-care workers to empower us, not give up on us. Those who care for us need to hear our concerns, fears, and frustrations. When we cannot speak, health-caregivers will have to ask us questions, pay close attention, and listen for unspoken messages.

> *We are what we repeatedly do.*
> *Excellence, then, is not an act, but a habit.*
> **Aristotle**

We stroke survivors need advocates within the system. I'm sure that some of my health-caregivers thought I was being difficult by asking questions and expressing my emotions, but those were the actions that helped me get well. It's easy to answer a stroke survivors' questions with the explanation that "it's hospital policy," but we deserve to know why the policy is what it is. We should be permitted to make our own decisions about our care unless we are simply unable to make them. We need understanding, encouragement, kindness, gentleness, and respect. We need psychological nourishment as much as our bodies need physical therapy.

Don't step on my courage

Health-care professionals—as well as our families and friends—must accept our perceptions because they constitute our reality. Ask us what we need. Avoid speaking for those of us who have aphasia except when absolutely necessary. Even then, ask permission to do so. Don't talk to us as if we are children or are stupid. Use eye contact and touch to display your concern and kindness. Don't interrupt us when we are trying to talk. It's hard enough to speak without having to say something twice. Don't forget that we can use gestures to speak.

Ask us what we think will help us heal. Don't make us feel more invisible than we already do by ignoring our needs and wants. Remind us how strong and resilient we are. An encouraging word to us can lift us up and help us make it through the day. Be careful of what you say. You can speak words that tend to rob us of the spirit to continue in this difficult time. Don't compare us to those who have had other illnesses because that denies us the opportunity to express our grief. Look beyond the obvious. Try to understand how we feel so that we feel safe enough to ask for what we need.

A Word to My Fellow Survivors

Whatever we cultivate in times of ease,
we gather as strength in times of change.

Jack Kornfield

Don't give up when you have been given a diagnosis of a brain attack. Even if you feel you don't have the power and conviction to carry on, trudge on. Become as independent as possible. Communication is the key no matter how you manage it. Families need to talk to each other regularly. Discuss what is working and what is not. Live in the present. Allow yourself to make mistakes. Smile often, even though you might not have anything you feel you can smile about. Enjoy each moment. Keep looking for the "silver lining" in everything that happens. Give yourself credit for the progress you have made. Treat yourself with respect all the time. Celebrate the large and small gains in your recovery. Heighten your awareness of the beauty in the world around you.

Become a savvy consumer of health care and get the information and support you need for yourself. Ask about a stroke support group in your area. Use the resources in this book to help you.

Stand up for yourself. Some of us have the tendency to see nurses and doctors as technicians who will make us well. In reality, we have to heal ourselves. Permit yourself to get through each day without feeling guilty about your emotions. Accentuate the positive and take responsibility for your own happiness. Living with a disability requires teamwork, planning, and hard work. Embrace challenges, because they will help you walk fearlessly toward your future.

I have learned that success is to be measured
not so much by the position that one has reached in life
as by the obstacles which he has overcome while trying to succeed.

Booker T. Washington

Surround yourself with people who believe in you, people you can rely on in an uncertain time. Even though we might be feeling scared and vulnerable, we must take a risk and set new goals for ourselves. Dare to dream.

Family-Centered Stroke Care

I have been a proponent of family-centered care for women in labor all my professional life. I have also been an advocate for the patient even when it wasn't fashionable. Advocacy is part of a health professional's job. What we say and do can affect the rest of a patient's life. The family-centered philosophy could be adapted to stroke care as a way for patients and their families and health-care providers to relate to each other. The stroke experience belongs not to caregivers, but to the patient's family and friends. They are the constants in the stroke survivor's life. Doctors, nurses, and therapists are only temporary players in the drama of recovery.

Traditionally, health-care professionals made most, if not all, decisions about care and treatments, while patients and families stood passively by. Often family members were regarded as unnecessary baggage who meant only trouble to staff members. Family-centered stroke care recognizes that families and friends play a vital role in the stroke victim's recovery, and it promotes the full participation of patients and their families in the planning, delivery, and evaluation of health-care services.

I needed my family and friends to help me survive the horrible onslaught of the brain attack when I couldn't speak for myself. My life would have been very different if I hadn't had a knowledgeable advocate in the ER who prodded and probed until she got information about tPA. But all patients, with or without an advocate, deserve to be supplied with unbiased information about stroke treatments in lay terms.

Introducing family-centered stroke care requires training doctors, nurses, and therapists to collaborate with patients and their families. Hospitals need to change their policies to invite input by families and friends of stroke survivors in the planning, implementation, and evaluation of stroke care. Shifting to family-centered stroke care is a complex task, but it is a necessity for all those who give and receive stroke care.

Principles of Family-Centered Care

- **Recognizes** the importance of families in ensuring the health and well-being of family members.

- **Promotes** sharing of information and collaboration among patients, families, and health-care staff.

- **Acknowledges** that emotional and social support is an integral component of health care.

- **Encourages** and facilitates patient-to-patient support.

- **Acknowledges** that families bring important strengths to their health-care experiences.

- **Empowers** individuals and families and fosters independence.

- **Supports** family caregiving and decision making.

- **Respects** the choices, values, beliefs, and cultural background of the patient and family.

- **Involves** patients and families in the planning, delivery, and evaluation of health-care services.

Stroke Survivor/ Family/ Professional Collaboration

This checklist can be used by groups setting up family-centered stroke care.

1. Are there formal and informal ways of ensuring effective family/patient/professional cooperation at all levels of care?

2. Are there both informal and formal ways of encouraging patient and family participation during planning and evaluation meetings?

3. Are the families and patients involved in planning representative of the demographics of the community that will be using the facility?

4. Are there ways to involve patients and families in training (inservice) programs?

5. Are there effective ways of obtaining information about patients from the patients and their family and friends and of disseminating relevant information back to them?

6. Are there inservice programs for professionals that build the skills necessary for family-centered care to work effectively?

Tips about Aphasia for Family and Friends

- Get the person's attention before you speak.

- At first use short, uncomplicated sentences, and write down words and repeat them.

- At first it may take 30 seconds or more for the stroke survivor to digest what you said.

- Speak in a natural voice. Talking more loudly won't help the person understand better.

- Maintain a natural, adult conversational manner.

- Minimize distractions like TV and radio.

- Always include the person with aphasia in your conversation.

- Don't interrupt or constantly correct the aphasic person.

- Encourage the use of gestures, pointing, and drawing.

- Allow the person plenty of time to talk, and praise any attempts to speak.

- Avoid being overprotective or speaking for the aphasic person.

- Involve the aphasic person in decision making.

- Don't talk to the aphasic person as if he were a child.

- Give the person time to grasp one idea before you move to another.

- A person with aphasia will follow conversations more easily if she is talking to one person.

APPENDIX
Effects of a Stroke

At least every minute of every day someone in the United States has a stroke. Every year 730,000 Americans will have a brain attack, and nearly 160,000 will die from it, making brain attacks the third leading cause of death in the United States after heart disease and cancer. An additional 500,000 people will have a mini-stroke. Approximately one-third of stroke survivors will have another stroke within five years, and the risk of recurrence increases about ten percent each year after the stroke.

Strokes are also a major cause of disability. Four million Americans are living with the effects of a stroke. About one-third have mild impairments, another third are moderately impaired, and the remainder are severely impaired.

Brain attacks aren't limited to older people. Twenty-eight percent of the victims are younger than 65. Men have a 19 percent greater risk of having a brain attack than women, although taking birth control pills and smoking cigarettes increases a woman's risk. Brain attacks are most common in the southeastern United States.

Strokes cost the United States about $30 billion every year. About $17 billion of that includes direct costs for hospitals, physicians, and therapists. The remainder consists of indirect costs such as lost productivity.

It is imperative that the public, physicians, and nonphysician emergency medical personnel know the symptoms of a stroke.

Symptoms of a Stroke

- Sudden numbness or weakness of a part of the face, an arm, or a leg, especially on one side of the body
- Sudden confusion, trouble speaking or understanding speech
- Sudden trouble seeing in one or both eyes
- Sudden, severe headache with no known cause

If you see or have any of these symptoms

CALL 911...

This call could save a life.

Treatment can be more effective if given quickly.

Every minute counts!

Stroke Survivors

Like cancer, stroke is no respecter of wealth, position, profession, or education. The following people have all survived, and in most cases recovered from, a stroke.

Mary Kay Ash, Businesswoman
Hoyt Axton, Musician
Ann Baxter, Actress
Barbara Bel Geddes, Actress
Winston Churchill, British Prime Minister
Claudette Colbert, Actress
Joseph Cotten, Actor
Bette Davis, Actress
Deng Xiao Ping, Chinese leader
Ram Dass, Spiritualist
Charles Dickens, Author
Kirk Douglas, Actor
Dale Evans, Actress
Federico Fellini, Director
President Gerald Ford
Robert Guillaume, Actor
Frederick Hart, Sculptor
Gene Kelly, Actor
Joseph Kennedy, Father of President John Kennedy
Rose Fitzgerald Kennedy, Mother of President John Kennedy
Burt Lancaster, Actor
Rod Laver, Tennis pro
Princess Margaret of England
Thelonius Monk, Musician
Patricia Neal, Actress
President Richard Nixon
Oscar Peterson, Musician
Della Reese, Actress
Ginger Rogers, Actress
Josef Stalin, Russian dictator
Mel Torme, Singer
President Woodrow Wilson

Types of Brain Attacks

Stroke is the term used for a lack of oxygen in the brain from an interruption in blood flow. Eighty percent of all brain attacks are of an ischemic nature (caused by a blood clot, or thrombus), and 20 percent are caused by a hemorrhage or bleeding.

Some new tests have recently been reported in the medical literature that can be used to determine which people can be helped by clot-breaking treatments. The battery of tests include cognitive tests combined with a rapid, readily available type of MRI (magnetic resonance) scan to identify which patients have salvageable brain tissue that would benefit from clot busters.

The American Heart Association developed criteria that patients must meet before thrombolytic treatment can begin. All three criteria must be met: Age 18 years or older; clinical diagnosis of ischemic stroke causing a measurable neurological deficit; time of symptom onset well-established and less than 180 minutes before thrombolytic treatment can begin.

People who have had an ischemic stroke may be prescribed medication to help prevent the formation of more clots. These medications include aspirin or other anticoagulants such as warfarin.

Components of Rehabilitation

- Cognitive exercises and computer-assisted strategies improve attention, memory, and executive function.
- Occupational, recreational, physical, and speech therapy address the deficits.
- Compensatory devices can improve cognitive function and compensate for deficits like short attention spans.
- Psychotherapy helps treat depression and loss of self-esteem.
- Behavioral modification addresses personality and behavioral effects and retrains social skills.
- Vocational rehabilitation supports employment and job coaching, as the return to work is one of the most significant outcomes of recovery.
- Alternative approaches (music, art, acupuncture, and nutritional support) have been helpful, but these interventions have not been systematically teste

Aphasia
Where have my words gone?

We may have all come on different ships,
but we're in the same boat now.
Martin Luther King

The ability to communicate with words is a human characteristic, and aphasia, or impaired communication, can affect every aspect of a person's life. Aphasia includes: impairment in speaking, trouble understanding speech, and difficulty with reading and writing. Intelligence is typically unimpaired.

Communication difficulties depend on where and how severely the brain was damaged. People with aphasia may have trouble conveying their thoughts because they have to formulate their thoughts and then find the words to express those thoughts. They may have trouble keeping in mind all the words they want to say at a particular time. They may be unable to understand what they hear because they have trouble keeping in their minds everything they heard until the speaker is finished. They may have difficulty using little words such as "the" and "of."

It is estimated by the National Aphasic Association that approximately 85,000 people become aphasic each year, most often from a stroke or head injury. About one million Americans currently have aphasia. Although there is no cure for aphasia or drugs to treat it, speech therapy and hard work can overcome many of the difficulties.

There are three types of aphasia: nonfluent, fluent, and global.

Characteristics of the Three Types of Aphasia

Nonfluent	Fluent	Global
effortful, hesitant, telegraphic speech	normal rate of speech without pauses	severe in all aspects of language performance
slow, incomplete sentences	reduction in ability to find a precise noun	very little speech
if severe, single-word vocabulary	use of nonsense words	difficulty understanding speech
reduction in vocabulary speaking and writing	difficulty understanding speech	

Approximately 80 percent of the studies of aphasia therapy concluded that therapy produces a significant improvement for most people if treatment begins early in the recovery process. Factors that influence the amount of improvement include the cause of the brain damage, the site of the damage, the extent of the injury, and the age, health, and motivation of the patient. Patients with a high level of social support make greater and faster improvements than patients without a support system. During recovery, the aphasic person's abilities to speak may fluctuate from day to day or even from morning to night.

Very few individuals with chronic aphasia will return to the job or position they had before the stroke. Exceptions are self-employed people or people in a position to make adjustments in the workplace. Speech therapy facilitates the return to work by targeting work-related communication skills. It has been reported that people who are motivated to return to gainful employment and are willing to make adaptations can go back to work regardless of the severity of their aphasia, but the return to work typically takes two to three years.

Resources

ADA Disability and Business Technical Assistance Centers
(800) 949-4232
www.adata.org

ADA Helpline- Equal Employment Opportunity Commission
Boston Area Office
JFK Federal Office Building, Room 475
Boston, MA 02203
(800) 669-4000

American Academy of Neurology
1080 Montreal Avenue
St. Paul, MN 55116
(651) 695-1940 (612) 623-8115
www.aan.com

American Academy of Physical Medicine and Rehabilitation
1 IBM Plaza, Suite 2500
Chicago, IL 60611
(312) 464-9700
www.aapmr.org
info@aapmr.org

American Association of Retired Persons (AARP)
601 E Street NW
Washington, DC 20049
(800) 424-3410
www.aarp.org

American Heart Association
7272 Greenville Avenue
Dallas, TX 75231
(214) 373-6300
(800) AHAUSA1
www.americanheart.org

American Occupational Therapy Association
4720 Montgomery Lane
Bethesda, MD 20814
(301) 652-2682
(800) 729-2682
www.aota.org

American Physical Therapy Association
1111 North Fairfax Street
Alexandria, VA 22314
(703) 684-2782
(800) 999-2782
www.apta.org

American Psychiatric Association
1400 K Street NW
Washington, DC 20005
(202) 682-6000
www.psych.org

American Speech-Language-Hearing Association
10801 Rockville Pike
Rockville, Maryland 20852
(888) 321-ASHA
www.asha.org
24 hours a day 7 days a
week automated information available
(800) 638-8255

ASHA Action Center
8:30am-5:00pm ET,
(800) 498-2071
TTY (301) 571-0457

BRAIN
Brain Resources and Information
Network
P.O. Box 13050
Silver Spring, MD 20911
(800) 352-9424

Center for Research in
Complementary and Alternative
Medicine for Stroke and
Neurological Disorders
Kessler Medical Rehabilitation Research
and Education Corporation (KMRREC)
1199 Pleasant Valley Way
West Orange, NJ 07052
(973) 731-3600
www.emdnj.edu/altmdweb

Courage Stroke Network
3915 Golden Valley Road
Golden Valley, MN 55422
(612) 588-0811

Depression Awareness, Recognition
and Treatment (D/ART)
National Institute of Mental Health
5600 Fishers Lane
Rockville, MD 20857
(800) 421-4211
www.nimh.nih.gov

IBM's National Support Center for
Persons with Disabilities
(800) 426-4832

International Society for Trauma
Stress Studies
60 Revere Drive, Suite 500
Northbrook, IL 60062
(847) 480-9028
www.istss.org

LinguiSystems, Inc.
3100 4th Avenue
East Moline, IL 61244
(800) PROIDEA
www.linguisystems.org

National Association of Social
Workers
750 1st Street NE
Washington, DC 20002
(800) 638-8799
www.socialworkers.org

National Aphasia Association
156 Fifth Avenue, Suite 707
New York, NY 10010
(8000 922-4622
www.aphasia.org

National Brain Injury Association
105 North Alfred Street
Alexandria, VA 22314
(703) 236-6000
(800) 444-6443
www.biausa.org

National Center for Post-Traumatic
Stress Disorder
VAM and ROC 116D
215 North Main Street
White Junction, VT 05009-0001
(802) 296-5132
www.ncptsd

National Easter Seal Society
230 West Monroe Street, Suite 1800
Chicago, IL 60606
(800) 221-6827
(312) 726-6200 (voice)
(312) 726-4258 (TDD)

Brain Attack

National Foundation of Depressive Illness
P.O. Box 2257
New York, NY 10116
(800) 239-1265

National Rehabilitation Information Center
1010 Wayne Avenue, Suite 800
Silver Spring, MD 20910
(800) 346-2742
www.NARI.com

National Rehabilitation Hospital Stroke Recovery Program
102 Irving Street NW
Washington, DC 20010-2921
(202) 877-1000
www.NRHREHAB.org

National Stroke Association
96 Inverness Drive East, Suite I
Englewood, CO 801222
(303) 649-9299
fax (303) 649-1328
(800) 787-6537
www.stroke.org

SAFE - Stroke Awareness For Everyone
8906 E. 96th St., #311
Fishers, IN 46038
317-585-9562
FAX 317-585-9563

Social Security Administration
PO Box 1756
Baltimore, MD 21235
(800) 772-1213
www.ssa.gov

Stroke Connection
American Heart Association
National Center
7272 Greenville Avenue
Dallas, TX 7523
(800) 553-6321
www.strokeassociation.org

US Department of Justice's ADA Information Line
(800) 514-0301
www.esdoj.gov/crt/ada/adahom1.html

US Equal Employment Opportunity Commission
(800) 669-4000
www.eeoc.gov

The VNA
11 Beacon Street, Suite 910
Boston, MA 02108
(888) 966-8773
www.VNAA.org

VNA HealthCare Services
1789 South Braddock Avenue
P.O. Box 82550
Pittsburgh, PA 15218
(800) 640-4VNA
http://www.vna-pgh.org/stroke.html

Internet Resources

American Heart Association	http://www.americanheart.org/
Aphasia Center of California	http://members.aol.com/rjelman/
Aphasia.com	http://www.aphasia.com
Aphasia Hope	http://www.aphasiahope.org
Aphasia- Language	http://faculty.washington.edu/chudler/lang.html
Courville Speech Therapy Site	http://members.aol.com/acourville/index.html
Kaiser Guidelines of Brain Imaging	http://www.strokeorg/Kaiser/Kaiser-imaging.html
National Institute of Deafness and Other Communication Disorders (NIDCD)	http://www.nidcd.nih.gov/
National Institute of Neurological Diseases and Stroke (NINDS)	http://www.ninds.nih.gov/
National Center for Post-Traumatic Stress Disorder	http://www.ncptsd.org/
Neurological Resource Center	http://www.span.com.au/nrc/stroke.html
Stroke	http://www.stroke.org
Stroke Journal	http://www.strokejournal.org
Stroke Matters	http://www.strokematters.com
University of Michigan Communicative Disorders Clinic	http://www.umich.edu/~comdis/geninf.html
We Media	http://www.wemedia.com
Stroke-TIA Organization	http://stroke-tia.org/
Agency for Healthcare Research and Quality	http://www.ahrq.gov/
American Physical Therapy Association	http://www.apta.org
Stroke Research and Treatment Center	http://www.fhsu.edu/stroke/

The Stroke Survivor's Bill of Rights

The period immediately after a stroke can be a frightening time for stroke survivors and their families. Sometimes a stroke survivor can understand everything that is going on around her or him, but is unable to speak or communicate due to paralysis and/or speech loss. The Stroke Survivor's Bill of Rights was written to educate, inform, support, and provide hope to stroke survivors and their families. The effects of stroke can be devastating and lead to depression and hopelessness. Hope is the essential ingredient for maximum recovery and rehabilitation. There is no such thing as false hope.

1. A stroke survivor has the right to a vigilant advocate – a family doctor and/or close family member or friend – to help interpret, question, and challenge her or his health care.

2. A stroke survivor has the right to expect courage from his or her family and friends – courage to be with her or him in the hospital, courage to speak the truth and challenge authority, courage to accept her or his new condition.

3. A stroke survivor has the right to health professionals who listen, encourage, hope, and join her or him as allies.

4. A stroke survivor has the right to be treated with respect. Even though, at first she or he may not be able to respond, chances are she or he understands what is being said.

5. A stroke survivor has the right to seek positive and creative practitioners, and to avoid anyone who makes negative or limiting prognoses or who puts her or him down in any way.

6. A stroke survivor has the right to take charge of her or his life. This means as soon as possible figuring out what she or he needs and becoming actively involved in her or his own care and rehabilitation.

7. A stroke survivor has the right to ask questions, challenge, and even object when necessary.

8. A stroke survivor has the right to be recognized as the leading expert about her or his own body.

9. A stroke survivor has the right to ask for help. By asking for help, she and he offers other people an opportunity for intimacy and collaboration. Whether asking for help for herself or himself personally, or for disabled people collectively, she or he gives others the opportunity to be their most human selves.

10. A stroke survivor has the right to seek out peers and allies, join with disability rights activists, and make a stink when necessary!

Bonnie Sherr Klein – *Out of the Blue" One Woman's Story of Stroke, Love, and Survival*

Glossary

ADL
> Activities of daily living such as eating, grooming, toileting, and dressing.

AIS
> Acute ischemic stroke.

Anoxia
> State of almost no oxygen delivery to a cell, resulting in low energy production and possible death of the cell.

Anticoagulant agents
> Drugs used in stroke prevention therapy to prevent blood clots from forming or growing. They interfere with the production of certain blood components necessary for clot formation.

Antithrombotics
> Type of anticoagulation therapy that prevents the formations of blood clots by inhibiting the coagulating actions of the blood protein thrombin.

Aphasia
> Impairment of the ability to use and comprehend words, usually acquired as a result of a stroke or other brain injury.

Apraxia
> Disorder of learned movement unexplained by deficits in strength, coordination, sensation or comprehension, generally caused by the damage to the areas of the brain responsible for voluntary movement.

Brain attack
> Term that more accurately describes the action and effect of a stroke on the brain.

CAT scan
> Series of cross-sectional x-rays of the head and brain that reveals the internal structure of the brain in precise detail.

Central stroke pain
> Also called central pain syndrome. Caused by damage to an area in the thalamus. The pain is a mixture of sensations, including heat and cold, burning, tingling, and numbness and sharp, stabbing and underlying aching pain.

Compensation
> The ability of an individual with impairments from stroke to perform a task (or tasks) using different modalities.

Brain Attack

Coumadin

Commonly used anticoagulant, also called warfarin.

CVA

Cerebrovascular accident. A term traditionally used for stroke. Stroke is no longer viewed as an accident.

Dysarthria

A language disorder characterized by difficulty with speaking or forming words.

Embolus

Free-roaming clot that usually forms in the heart.

Embolic stroke

Stroke resulting from the blockage of an artery by a blood clot (embolus).

Hypoxia

Lack of oxygen.

Hemiparesis

Weakness on one side of the body.

Incidence

The frequency with which new and recurrent cases of a specific disease occur during a certain period of time in a quantitatively undefined population (e.g., annual stroke incidence is the USA is 730,000).

Incidence rate

The number of new and recurrent cases of a disease that occur during a specified period of time per a defined number of individuals in a reference population (e.g., annual stroke incidence rate in African-Americans is 288 per 100.000).

Infarct

The immediate area of brain-cell death caused by the stroke. When the brain cells in the infarct die, they release chemicals that set off a chain reaction that endangers brain cells in a larger surrounding area.

Interdisciplinary treatment

Treatment delivered to a patient by two or more medical or rehabilitative disciplines working collaboratively.

Ischemia

An interruption or blockage of blood flow.

Left hemisphere

The half of the brain that controls the actions of the right side of the body, as well as analytic abilities such as calculating, speaking, and writing.

Occupational therapist

Therapist who focuses on helping stroke survivors rebuild skills in daily living activities, such as bathing, toileting, and dressing.

Physiatrist

Medical doctor who specializes in rehabilitation.

Physical therapist

Healthcare professional who specializes in maximizing a stroke survivor's mobility and independence in order to improve major motor and sensory impairments in walking, balance, and coordination.

Prosody

Rhythm and timing of speech.

Rehabilitation nurse

Nurse who coordinates the medical support needs of stroke survivors throughout rehabilitation.

Recreational therapist

Therapist who helps to modify activities that the stroke survivor enjoyed before the stroke or introduces new ones.

Psychiatrist/psychologist

Specialist who helps stroke survivors adjust to the emotional challenges and new circumstances of their lives.

Social worker

Counselor of psychological needs, including sexuality.

SLP

Speech-language pathologist: a professional educated in the development and disorders of human communication.

Stenosis

Severe narrowing of an artery.

Stroke

Sudden interruption of blood flow to a part of the brain that kills cells within the area. Body functions controlled by the affected area may be impaired or lost.

Thrombolytic agents

Acute interventional drugs that break up or dissolve stroke-causing clots.

Thromboembolism

Embolus that breaks away from a clot in one vessel to become lodged in another vessel.

Brain Attack

Thrombosis

Clotting of blood within a vessel.

tPA

Synthetic form of tissue plasminogen activator. This drug is a thrombolytic agent used to dissolve blood clots. Given intravenously, it is the only drug currently approved by the Food and Drug Administration for treating acute ischemic stroke.

Transesophageal echogram

This procedure is performed to evaluate the valves and chambers of the heart.

Vocational therapist

A specialist who evaluates work-related abilities of people with disabiities.

Bibliography

To Read More about Strokes. Aphasia, Apraxia, and Feelings

Adams, Kathleen. *Journal to the Self: 22 Paths to Personal Growth*, Warner Books, 1990.

Adams, Harold P. *Guidelines for Thrombolytic Therapy for Acute Stroke: A Supplement to the Guidelines for the Management for Patients with Ischemic Stroke*, American Heart Association, Dallas, TX, 1996.

Allen, John G. *Coping with Trauma: A Guide to Self-Understanding*, American Psychiatric Press, 1995.

American Heart Association. *Caring for a Person with Aphasia.* 1994, 800/553-6321. www.americanheart.org.

American Heart Association. *How Stroke Affects Behavior*, 1994, 800/553-6321. www.americanheart.org.

Ancowitz, Arthur. *The Stroke Book*, Thorndike Press, 1994.

Bauby, Jean-Dominique. *The Diving Bell and the Butterfly*, Vintage, 1998.

Bergquist, W.H. and Kobylinski. *Stroke Survivors*, Jossey-Bass, Inc., San Francisco, CA, 1994.

Bolen, Jean Shinoda. *Close to the Bone*, Touchstone, 1996.

Boone, Daniel. *An Adult Has Aphasia* (5th ed.), ProEd Publishers, Inc., Austin, TX, 1984.

Briskin, Alan. *The Stirring of the Soul in the Work Place,* Berrett-Koehler Publisher, 1998.

Broida, H. *Coping with Stroke: Communication of Brain Injured Adults*, College Hill Press. Houston, TX.

Byng, Sally; Gilpin, Sue; Ireland, Chris; and Parr, Susie, *Talking About Aphasia: Living with Loss of Language*, Taylor & Francis, 1997.

DeSalvo, Louise. *Writing as a Way of Healing*, Beacon Press, 2000.

Dominic O'Brien, *Learn to Remember: Practical Techniques and Exercises to Improve Your Memory,* Chronicle Books, San Franciso, 2000.

Ewing, S.S. and Pfalzgraf. *Pathways: Moving Beyond Stroke and Aphasia*, Wayne Sate University Press. Detroit, MI. 301/577-6120.

Golman, Daniel. *Emotional Intelligence*, Bantam, 1993.

Herman, Judith. *Trauma and Recovery*, Basic Books, 1993.

Hickley, Jacqueline. *What is it Like to Have Trouble Communicating?*, Interactive Therapeutic, Inc., Stow, OH, www.interactivetherapy.com.

Jacob, L., et al. *Adult Aphasia: Understanding the Disability* (3rd ed.), Department pf Communication Disorders, Youville Hospital and Rehabilitation Center, Cambridge, MA, 617/876-4344, 1994.

Jones, Cynthia and Lorman, Janis. *Aphasia: A Guide for Patient and Family*, Interactive Therapeutics, Inc., Stow, OH, www.interactivetherapy.com.

Jones, Cynthia and Lorman, Janis. *Apraxia: A Guide for Patient and Family*, Interactive Therapeutics, Inc., Stow, OH, www.interactivetherapy.com.

Jones, Cynthia and Lorman, Janis. *Dysarthria: A Guide for Patient and Family*, Interactive Therapeutics, Inc., Stow, OH, www.interactivetherapy.com.

Lyon, Jon G. *Coping with Aphasia*, Singular Publishing Group, Inc., 1988. **800/521- 8545.**

Kaufman, Beth. *Apraxia Treatment Manual*, Imaginart International, Bisbee, AZ, 800/828-1376.

Klein, Bonnie Sherr. *Out of the Blue: One Woman's Story of Stroke, Love and Survival*, Wild Canyon Press, 2000.

Knight, Marla. *Right Brain Stroke: A Guide for Patient and Family*, Interactive Therapeutics, Inc., Stow, OH, www.interactivetherapy.com.

Knox. David. *Portrait of Aphasia*, Wayne State University, Detroit, MI, 1971.

McCullough, Michael, Everret Worthington & Steven Sandage. *To Forgive Is Human: How to Put Your Past in the Past*, Intervarsity Press, 1997.

McCrum, Robert. *My Year Off: Recovering Life After a Stroke*, Norton, 1998.

Miller, Emmett. *Deep Healing: The Essence of Mind/Body Medicine*, Hay House, 1997.

The Silent Minority: *The Patient with Aphasia,*

Sarno, Martha Taylor,*The Fifth Annual James C. Hemphill Lecture*, National Aphasia Association, 156 Fifth Avenue, Suite 707, New York, NY 10010,1986. (800) 922-4622

National Stroke Association.*Living at Home after Your Stroke*, National Stroke Association, Englewood, CO,1994, 800/787-6537, www.stroke.org.

Neal, Patricia. *As I Am: An Autobiography*, Simon and Schuster, 1988.

Pennebaker, James W. *Opening Up: The Healing Power of Confiding in Others*, William Morrow & Co., 1990.

Pert, Candace. *Molecules of Emotions: The Science Behind Mind-Body Medicine*, Touchstone, 1999.

Sacks, Oliver. *The Man Who Mistook His Wife for a Hat*, Touchstone Books, 1989.

Sarno, Martha Taylor. *The Silent Minority: The Patient with Aphasia*, The Fifth Annual James C. Hemphill Lecture, National Aphasia Association, 1986, 800/922-4622.

Sarton, May. *After the Stroke*, Norton, 1998.

Schaef, Anne Wilson. *Living in Process: Basic Truths for Living the Path of the Soul*, Ballantine Wellspring,1999.

Tanner, Dennis C. *The Family Guide to Surviving Stroke and Communication Disorders*, Allyn & Bacon, Needham Heights, MA, 1999, 800/278-3525, www.abacon.com

Wallace, Gloriajean. *Adult Aphasia Rehabilitation*, Butterworth-Heinemann Medical, 1996.

Weiner. Lee. *Recovering at Home After a Stroke*, Body Press, 1994.